AQA A2

Physical Education

Carl Atherton Symond Burrows Sue Young

Philip Allan Updates, an imprint of Hodder Education, an Hachette UK company, Market Place, Deddington, Oxfordshire OX15 0SE

Orders
Bookpoint Ltd, 130 Milton Park, Abingdon, Oxfordshire OX14 4SB
tel: 01235 827720
fax: 01235 400454
e-mail: uk.orders@bookpoint.co.uk

Lines are open 9.00 a.m.–5.00 p.m., Monday to Saturday, with a 24-hour message answering service. You can also order through the Philip Allan Updates website:
www.philipallan.co.uk

ISBN 978-1-84489-644-8

Impression number 5 4 3 2 1
Year 2013 2012 2011 2010 2009

Printed in Italy.

Hachette UK's policy is to use papers that are natural, renewable and recyclable products and made from wood grown in sustainable forests. The logging and manufacturing processes are expected to conform to the environmental regulations of the country of origin.

P01353

Contents

Introduction ... vii

Unit 3 Optimising performance and evaluating contemporary issues within sport

Applied physiology to optimise performance

Chapter 1 Energy sources and systems
Adenosine triphosphate ... 2
Anaerobic energy systems: the ATP-PC system ... 4
Anaerobic energy systems: the lactate anaerobic system ... 5
The aerobic system ... 6
The energy continuum ... 8

Chapter 2 Fatigue and recovery
Causes of fatigue ... 11
Offsetting fatigue ... 13
The recovery process ... 13

Chapter 3 What makes a successful endurance performance?
Significance of maximum oxygen consumption in sporting performance ... 18
Evaluation of VO_2 max ... 20
Onset of blood lactate accumulation (OBLA) ... 21

Chapter 4 Structure and function of muscles
Control of muscular contraction ... 24
Types of muscle fibre ... 24
The sliding filament hypothesis ... 25
The motor unit ... 27

Chapter 5 Sports supplements
Sports supplements ... 29
Ergogenic aids ... 31
Preparing the body for training and performance ... 32

Chapter 6 Specialised training

Altitude training ... 35
Plyometrics ... 35
Proprioceptive neuromuscular facilitation (PNF) ... 36
Periodisation ... 37
Lactate sampling ... 39
Respiratory exchange ratio (RER) ... 39

Chapter 7 Sports injuries

Prevention and rehabilitation ... 42
DOMS ... 43

Chapter 8 Mechanics of movement

Linear motion ... 45
Newton's laws of motion ... 45
The measurements used in linear motion ... 46
Force ... 51
Impulse ... 56
Projectile motion ... 57
Angular motion ... 59

Psychological aspects that optimise performance

Chapter 9 Individual influences on the sports performer

Personality ... 66
Trait theory ... 66
Social learning theory ... 69
The interactionist approach ... 70
Achievement motivation ... 71
Attitudes ... 72
Aggression in sport ... 76

Chapter 10 Playing in a team

Team dynamics ... 80
Cohesion and coordination within the team ... 81
Leadership ... 85

Chapter 11 Emotional control of sporting performance

Confidence in sport ... 89
Self-efficacy theory ... 89
Goal setting in sport ... 92
Anxiety and stress in sport ... 93

The relationship between arousal and performance ... 101
Social facilitation and inhibition ... 106
Attribution theory ... 109

Evaluating contemporary influences

Chapter 12 World Games and supporting the development of elite performers

Key characteristics of World Games ... 112
The impact of World Games events ... 113
Sport England's sport development continuum ... 114
Talent identification and development programmes ... 116
Organisational support structure ... 117
Sport England ... 117
Other home country sports councils ... 120
UK Sport ... 121
National governing bodies of sport ... 130
The British Olympic Association (BOA) ... 132
Sports Coach UK ... 133
Funding of elite amateur sports performers in the UK ... 134

Chapter 13 The origins of modern-day sport and associated sporting ethics

The development of rational recreation ... 136
The formation of national governing bodies of sport ... 143
Rationalisation of sport: case studies ... 144
Amateurism and professionalism ... 146
The contract to compete ... 148
The Olympic ideal ... 148

Chapter 14 Sport, deviance and the law

Violence among sports performers ... 152
Violence among spectators: football hooliganism ... 154
Drug taking in sport ... 156
Sport and the law ... 160

Chapter 15 Sport and commercialisation

The relationships between sport, the media and business ... 163
Commercialisation ... 163
The media ... 166
Media technology ... 168
Sports technology: case studies ... 169

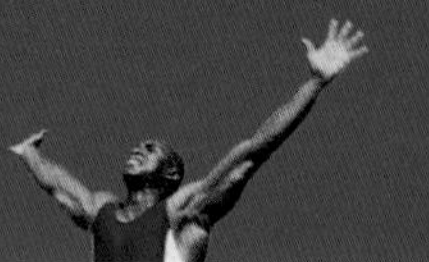

Unit 4 Optimising practical performance in a competitive situation

Chapter 16 Coursework

Section A: Practical performance 172

Section B: Observation, analysis and critical evaluation 173

Section C: Application of knowledge and understanding to optimise performance 174

Answers

Tasks to tackle 176

Practice makes perfect 186

Index 200

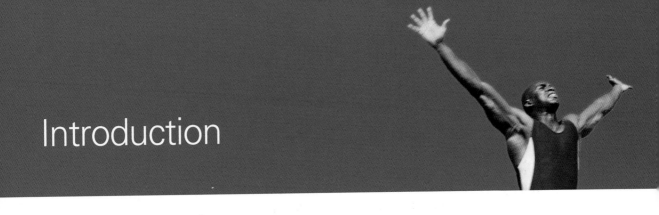

Introduction

About this book

This textbook is written for students following the AQA A2 specification in PE.

The topics, which appear in the same order as in the specification, are explained clearly. Links to practical examples will help you to relate this theory to your own sporting experiences.

Each chapter contains a number of features designed to aid your understanding of the requirements of the AQA A2 PE course:

- **Aims and objectives.** Each chapter begins with a clear outline of the subject matter and main topics covered.
- **Key terms.** Concise definitions of important terms are given throughout the book. A clear understanding of the key terms will reduce your chances of producing irrelevant answers in your exam, and hopefully earn more marks.
- **Top tips.** The authors use their considerable experience as teachers and examiners to provide useful pointers to help your exam performance and to avoid potential pitfalls. These tips include topic-specific help as well as tips for improving exam performance.
- **Tasks to tackle.** It is important to check your understanding of the topics covered in this book on a regular basis. 'Tasks to tackle' have been set to help you do this. Once you have attempted the tasks, check your answers against those provided at the back of the book.
- **Practice makes perfect.** These exam-style questions are designed to further assess your learning and understanding. Complete these questions as you progress through each main topic area (try to do this without referring to the text answers or your own notes). Solutions are provided at the back of the book for you to check your understanding.

Online resource

An online resource provides a selection of exam-style questions for you to tackle. These are followed by suggested answers and examiner comments. It also includes a worksheet with answers and some frequently asked questions to give you an idea of what to expect in your final exam. To access this resource, go to www.hodderplus.co.uk/philipallan.

The specification

The AQA A2 PE course involves two units, building on Units 1 and 2 already completed for AS. With the AS counting for 50% of the overall A-level, the final two units account for the other 50%. A2 theoretical study is contained in Unit 3, which is entitled **'Optimising performance and evaluating contemporary issues within sport'**. This is assessed in a 2-hour written exam, which is worth 84 marks in total. The exam has three parts to it, which are equally weighted (i.e. worth 28 marks each). The three sections are:

- **Section A** Applied physiology to optimise performance
- **Section B** Psychological aspects that optimise performance
- **Section C** Evaluating contemporary influences

This book follows the specification order outlined above and contains all the subject content necessary to help you achieve success in the final exam.

A2 coursework is contained in Unit 4, which is entitled **'Optimising practical performance in a competitive situation'**. This will involve you 'performing' one role from the following:

- practical performer
- coach
- official

This coursework is worth 20% of your overall A-level. In addition to actually performing this role, you will need to complete a written or verbal analysis and evaluation of your chosen role, identify any weaknesses you have in relation to an elite performer, and suggest causes of such weaknesses and appropriate corrective measures for them. Such corrective measures will need to be drawn from across the specification. This book contains some examples of different roles to help you understand how you will be assessed in your chosen role. Chapter 16 contains additional guidance.

Maximising your performance

Keeping up to date

This textbook contains many examples to illustrate the physiological, psychological, historical and socio-cultural points made. However, in the rapidly changing world of contemporary sport, it is important to keep as up to date as possible. New organisations and initiatives are being developed all the time to enhance the reputation of Great Britain as an excellent sporting nation. The best way to keep up to date is to visit the website addresses of the key organisations identified in the PHED3 specification. Reading good broadsheet newspapers such as the *Guardian* and the *Independent* is also an excellent way of keeping abreast of the ever-changing world of twenty-first century sport.

In the exam

The key elements that can help you to identify the skills being tested in a particular question and to answer that question effectively are:

- trigger words
- mark allocations
- knowledge of key terms

Trigger words

Specific trigger words are used in AQA A-level PE examinations. It is important that you understand the meaning of each of these words and that you answer the question appropriately.

- **Define/explain** — requires you to develop an answer that illustrates clearly your understanding of a word or term
- **Discuss** — this is more likely to appear at A2 than AS, and it requires you to describe and evaluate, putting forward various opinions or alternative viewpoints on a topic
- **Compare/contrast** — point out similarities and differences

Mark allocations

The first question in each of the three sections of the Unit 3 examination — physiology/biomechanics, sports psychology and contemporary issues — is compulsory and you must answer them. These questions are worth 14 marks each. They will be awarded marks according to banded statements. Once your answer has been marked, the examiner will place it into one of the band ranges given in the mark scheme. The examiner is looking for an answer that:

- addresses all parts of the question
- makes a variety of relevant points
- is written in continuous prose with few errors in spelling, punctuation and grammar, and uses correct technical language

It is therefore important to structure your work and to pay attention to your style of writing.

All other questions are worth 7 marks. You have to answer two questions from three *in each section.*

Key terms

Build up your own glossary of key terms as you progress through the topics in this textbook. This should consist of the words and phrases stipulated in the Unit 3 specification. Building up your own glossary will help when you come to revise, because you will have a few pages of key terms defined clearly in ways that are meaningful to you. These will help when you are asked to define or give the meaning of something.

Tips for exam success

- Read the question carefully, at least twice. On the second read through, highlight key words to help you focus on the key requirements to achieve the mark allocation.
- Answer the question set, not one you wish was set and have revised for. Relevance is the key to success. Irrelevant answers will earn no points.
- Avoid repetition. Try to ensure that any points you make are sufficiently different (and relevant) to achieve marks. Students often make the number of points required by the mark allocation, thinking they will score maximum marks. This may not be the case if a point is repeated. Several alternatives are often contained within one marking point and each mark scheme point can only be awarded once.

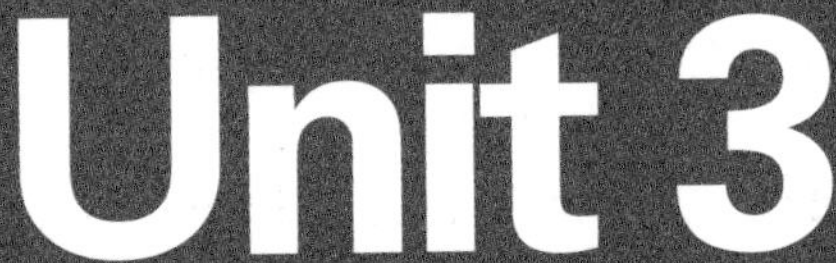

Unit 3

Optimising performance and evaluating contemporary issues within sport

- Applied physiology to optimise performance
- Psychological aspects that optimise performance
- Evaluating contemporary influences

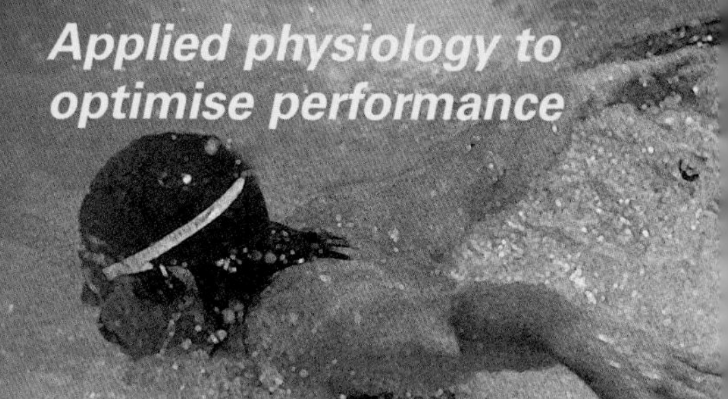

Chapter 1 Energy sources and systems

Applied physiology to optimise performance

What you need to know

By the end of this chapter you should be able to:

- identify which energy source is used according to the intensity and duration of an exercise
- state where these sources are located in the body
- understand how ATP is released and regenerated
- understand the ATP-PC system and the lactic acid system and their use in sporting situations
- understand the different stages of the aerobic system, to include glycolysis, the Krebs cycle, the electron transport chain and the role of the mitochondria
- understand the lactate threshold through the energy continuum

We need a constant supply of energy so that we can perform everyday tasks such as tissue repair and body growth. When we exercise we need energy for muscle contraction in order to produce movements such as running, jumping, catching and throwing. The more exercise we do the more energy is required. This chapter looks at how this energy is provided and how the body caters for different types of exercise, from the 100 metres where energy is required very quickly, to the marathon where energy needs to be provided for a long period of time. The *intensity* and *duration* of an activity play an important role in the way in which energy is provided.

Adenosine triphosphate

Adenosine triphosphate, more commonly referred to as ATP, is the only usable form of energy in the body. The energy we derive from the foods that we eat, such as carbohydrates, has to be converted into ATP before the potential energy in them can be used. As its name suggests, an ATP molecule consists of adenosine and three (tri) phosphates (Figure 1.1).

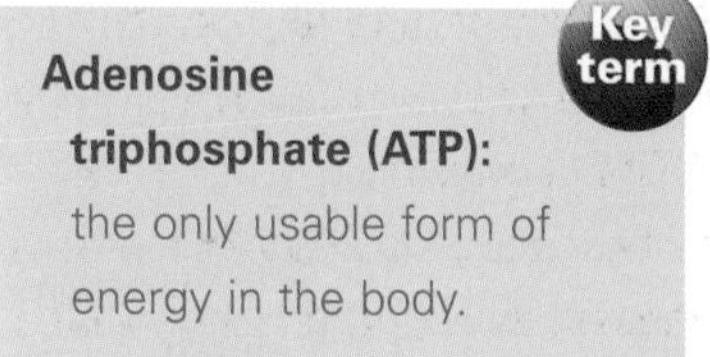

Key term

Adenosine triphosphate (ATP): the only usable form of energy in the body.

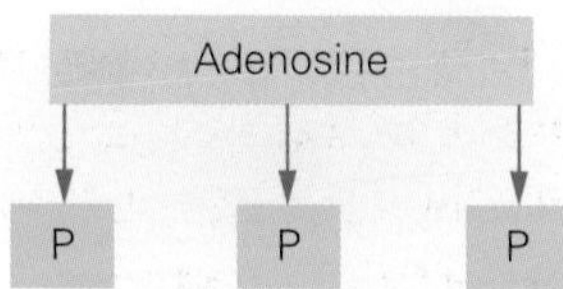

Figure 1.1 An ATP molecule

The release of ATP

Energy is released from ATP by breaking down the bonds that hold this compound together (Figure 1.2).

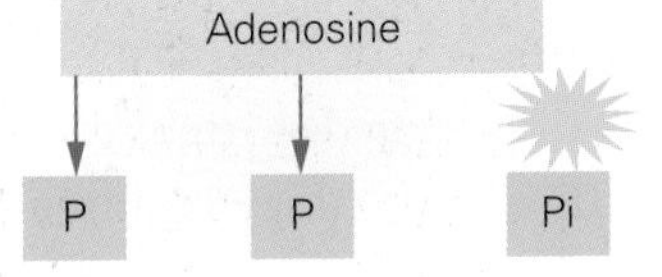

Figure 1.2 Energy is released when the molecule is broken down

Enzymes are used to break down compounds, and in this instance ATP-ase is the enzyme used to break down ATP into ADP (adenosine diphosphate) + **Pi** (Figure 1.3).

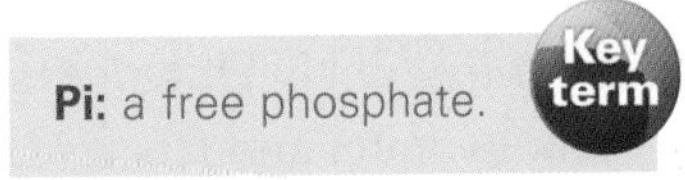

Pi: a free phosphate.

This type of reaction is an **exothermic reaction** because energy is released. A reaction that needs energy to work is called an **endothermic reaction**. Regenerating or resynthesising ATP from ADP + Pi is an endothermic reaction.

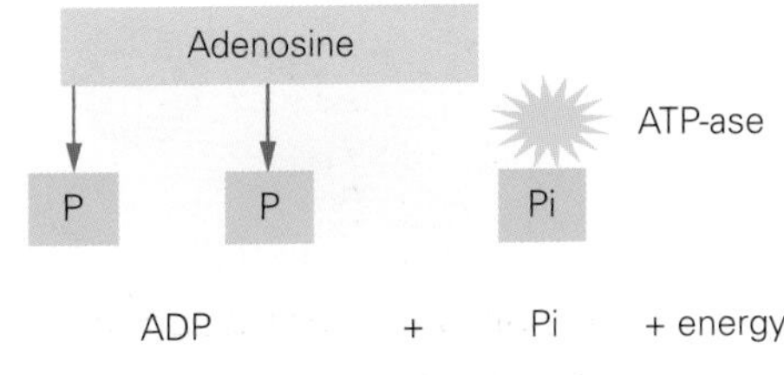

Figure 1.3 ATP → ADP + Pi + energy

The regeneration of ATP

As there is only a limited store of ATP within the muscle fibres, it is used up very quickly (in about 2–3 seconds) and therefore needs to be replenished immediately. There are three energy systems that regenerate ATP:

- the ATP-PC system
- the lactate anaerobic system
- the aerobic system

Each energy system is suited to a particular type of exercise depending on the intensity and duration and whether oxygen is present. The higher the intensity of the activity the more the individual will rely on anaerobic energy production from either the ATP-PC or lactate anaerobic systems. The lower the intensity and the longer the duration of the activity, the more the individual will use the aerobic system.

Sources of energy to replenish ATP

Each of the above energy systems uses fuels for ATP regeneration. These fuels can be derived from either a chemical or a food source.

Phosphocreatine is a chemical produced naturally by the body and used to regenerate ATP in the first 10 seconds of intense exercise. It is easy to break down and is stored within the muscle cells but its stores are limited. This is the fuel for the ATP-PC system.

Carbohydrates are stored as **glycogen** in the muscles and the liver, and converted into glucose during exercise. During high-intensity anaerobic exercise, glycogen can be broken down without the presence of oxygen (in the lactate anaerobic system), but it is broken down much more effectively during aerobic work when oxygen is present (in the aerobic system).

Fats are stored as triglycerides and converted to free fatty acids when required. At rest, two-thirds of our energy requirements can be achieved through the breakdown of fatty acids. This is because fat can produce more energy per gram than glycogen. Fat contains a lot of carbon, which is why it gives us so much energy. It is the secondary energy fuel for low-intensity, aerobic work such as jogging, but has to be used in combination with glycogen due to its hydrophobic quality (low water solubility), which inhibits fat metabolism.

Protein, in the form of amino acids, provides the source of approximately 5–10% of energy used during exercise. It tends to be oxidised when stores of glycogen are low.

Carbohydrates and fats are the main energy providers, and the intensity and duration of exercise plays a major role in determining which of these are used. The breakdown of fats to free fatty acids requires around 15% more oxygen than is required to break down glycogen, so during high-intensity exercise when oxygen is in limited supply, glycogen will be the preferred source of energy. Fats, therefore, are the favoured fuel at rest and during long, endurance-based activities.

Stores of glycogen are much smaller than stores of fat and it is important during prolonged periods of exercise not to deplete glycogen stores. Some glycogen needs to be conserved for later when the intensity could increase, for example during the last kilometre of a marathon.

Top tip

Questions on energy sources have been popular and tend to be related to specific performers — for example, the energy sources of a triathlete are carbohydrates, fats and proteins, due to the duration of the event.

Anaerobic energy systems: the ATP-PC system

Phosphocreatine (PC) is an energy-rich phosphate compound found in the sarcoplasm of the muscles, and is readily available. Its rapid availability is important for providing contractions of high power, such as in the 100 m or in a short burst of intense activity during a longer game (for example, a serve followed by a sprint to reach the return and perform a winning volley in tennis, or a fast break in basketball). However, there is only enough PC to last for up to 10 seconds and it can only be replenished when the intensity of the activity is sub-maximal.

The ATP-PC system regenerates ATP when the enzyme creatine kinase detects high levels of ADP. It breaks down the phosphocreatine to phosphate and creatine, releasing energy:

phosphocreatine (PC) → phosphate (Pi) + creatine (C) + energy

Key term

Phosphocreatine (PC): an energy-rich phosphate compound found in the sarcoplasm of the muscles.

This energy is then used to convert ADP to ATP. This breaking down of PC to release energy which is then used to convert ADP into ATP is a **coupled reaction** — for every molecule of

PC broken down there is enough energy released to create one molecule of ATP. This means that the system is not very efficient but it does have the advantage of not producing fatiguing by-products and its use is important in delaying the onset of the lactic anaerobic system.

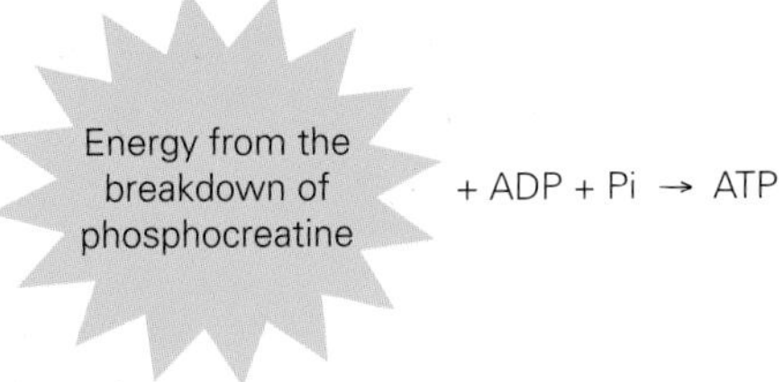

Figure 1.4 The ATP-PC system

Table 1.1 Advantages and disadvantages of the ATP-PC system

Advantages of the ATP-PC system	Disadvantages of the ATP-PC system
ATP can be regenerated rapidly using the ATP-PC system. Phosphocreatine stores can be regenerated quickly (30 secs = 50% replenishment and 3 mins = 100%). There are no fatiguing by-products. It is possible to extend the time the ATP-PC system can be utilised through use of creatine supplementation.	There is only a limited supply of phosphocreatine in the muscle cell, i.e. it can only last for 10 seconds. Only one molecule of ATP can be regenerated for every molecule of PC. PC regeneration can only take place in the presence of oxygen (i.e. when the intensity of the exercise is reduced).

Tasks to tackle 1.1

Think of three sporting examples in which the ATP-PC system would be the predominant method of regenerating ATP.

Anaerobic energy systems: the lactate anaerobic system

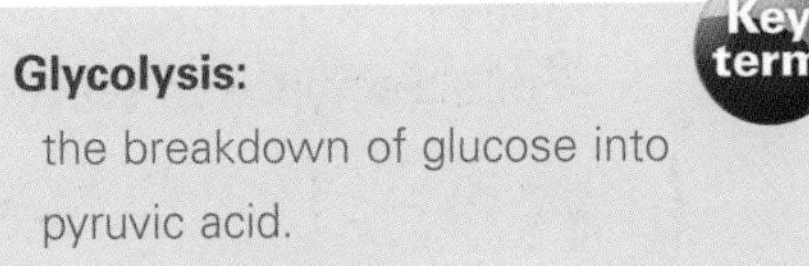

Glycolysis: the breakdown of glucose into pyruvic acid.

Once PC is depleted (at around 10 seconds) the lactate anaerobic system takes over and regenerates ATP from the breakdown of glucose. Glucose is stored in the muscles and liver as glycogen. Before glycogen can be used to provide energy to make ATP it has to be converted to glucose. This process is called **glycolysis** and the lactate anaerobic system is sometimes referred to as **anaerobic glycolysis**, due to the absence of oxygen.

In a series of reactions, the glucose molecule is broken down into two molecules of pyruvic acid, which is then converted to lactic acid by the enzyme lactate dehydrogenase, because oxygen is not available. The main enzyme responsible for the anaerobic breakdown of glucose is phosphofructokinase (PFK), activated by low levels of phosphocreatine. The energy released from the breakdown of each molecule of glucose is used to make two molecules of ATP.

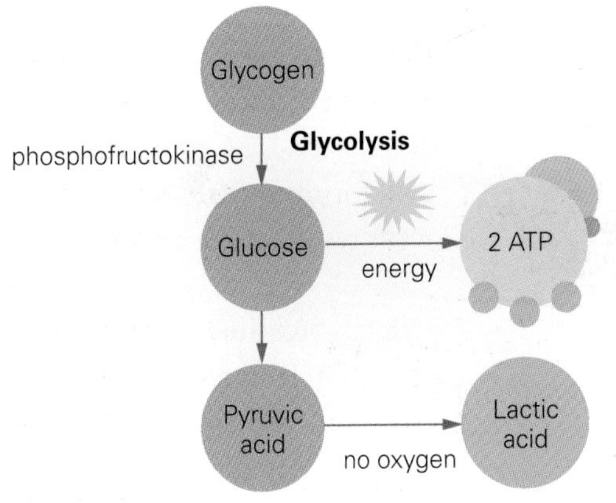

Figure 1.5 The lactate anaerobic system

The lactate anaerobic system provides energy for high-intensity activities lasting up to 3 minutes but peaking at 1 minute, for example running 400 m.

Table 1.2 Advantages and disadvantages of the lactate anaerobic system

Advantages of the lactate anaerobic system	Disadvantages of the lactate anaerobic system
ATP can be regenerated quite quickly due to very few chemical reactions being required. In the presence of oxygen, lactic acid can be converted back into liver glycogen or used as a fuel through oxidation into carbon dioxide and water. The process comes into use for a sprint finish (i.e. to produce an extra burst of energy).	Lactic acid is the by-product of this system. The accumulation of lactic acid in the body denatures enzymes and prevents them increasing the rate at which chemical reactions take place. Only a small amount of energy can be released from glycogen under anaerobic conditions (5% as opposed to 95% under aerobic conditions).

The aerobic system

This system breaks down glucose into carbon dioxide and water which, in the presence of oxygen, is much more efficient. The complete oxidation of glucose can produce up to 38 molecules of ATP and has three stages:

1 **Glycolysis.** This process is the same as anaerobic glycolysis (see above) but occurs in the presence of oxygen. Lactic acid is not produced and the pyruvic acid is converted into a compound called acetyl-coenzyme-A (acetyl-CoA).

2 **Krebs cycle.** Once the pyruvic acid diffuses into the matrix of the mitochondria (the powerhouses of muscle cells) forming acetyl-CoA, a complex cycle of reactions occurs in a process known as the Krebs cycle. Here, acetyl-CoA combines with oxaloacetic acid, forming citric acid. The reactions that occur result in the production of two molecules of ATP, as well as carbon dioxide, which is breathed out, and hydrogen, which is taken to the electron transport chain.

3 **Electron transport chain.** Hydrogen is carried to the electron transport chain by hydrogen carriers. This occurs in the cristae of the mitochondria. The hydrogen splits

Key term

Krebs cycle: a series of cyclical chemical reactions that use oxygen and take place in the matrix of the mitochondria.

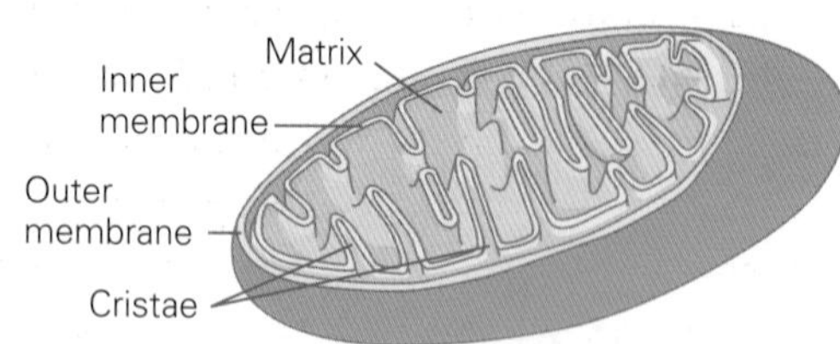

Figure 1.6 A cross-section through a mitochondrion

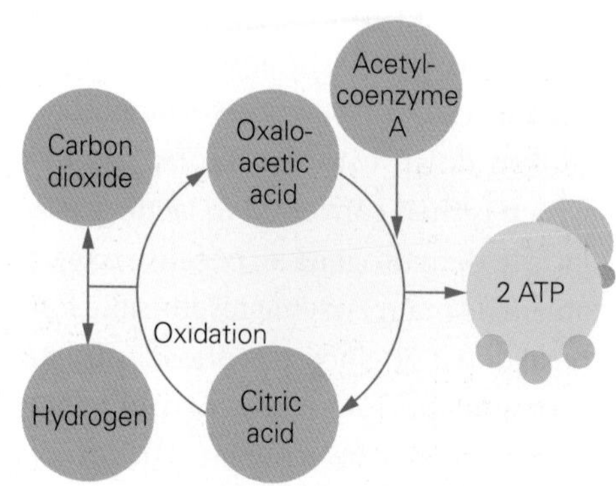

Figure 1.7 The Krebs cycle

into hydrogen ions and electrons and these are charged with potential energy. The hydrogen ions are oxidised to form water, while the electrons provide the energy to resynthesise ATP. Throughout this process, 34 ATP molecules are formed.

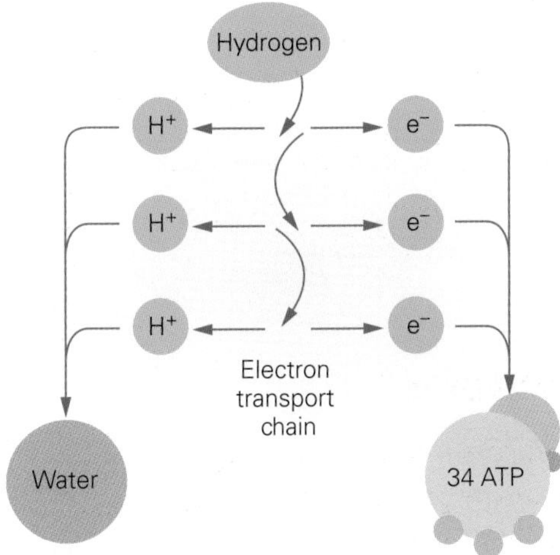

Figure 1.8 The electron transport chain

Beta oxidation

Fats can also be used as an energy source in the aerobic system. The Krebs cycle and the electron transport chain can metabolise fat as well as carbohydrate to produce ATP. First, the fat is broken down into glycerol and free fatty acids. These fatty acids then undergo a process called beta oxidation whereby they are broken down in the mitochondria to generate acetyl-CoA, which is the entry molecule for the Krebs cycle. From this point on, fat metabolism follows the same path as carbohydrate (glycogen) metabolism. More ATP can be made from one molecule of fatty acids than from one molecule of glycogen, which is why in long-duration exercise fatty acids will be the predominant energy source.

Table 1.3 Advantages and disadvantages of the aerobic system

Advantages of the aerobic system	Disadvantages of the aerobic system
More ATP can be produced than by anaerobic systems – 38 ATP molecules from the complete breakdown of each glucose molecule. There are no fatiguing by-products (only carbon dioxide and water). There are lots of glycogen and triglyceride stores, so exercise can last for a long time.	This is a complicated system so cannot be used straight away. It takes a while for enough oxygen to become available to meet the demands of the activity and ensure glycogen and fatty acids are completely broken down. Fatty acid transportation to muscles is low and fatty acids require 15% more oxygen to break them down than glycogen.

Top tip

Make sure you have a basic overview of each energy system and can identify when each system is used. If the question asks for the main energy system used, then just give the relevant one — if you name all the systems, no marks will be awarded.

Figure 1.9 shows a summary of ATP regeneration from the complete breakdown of glycogen.

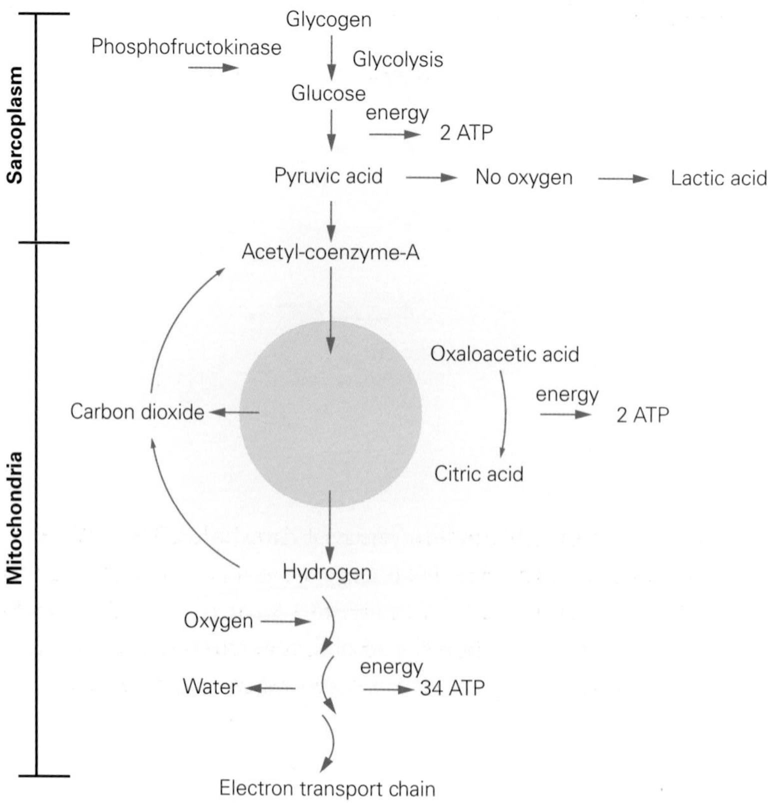

Figure 1.9 Summary of the aerobic system

The energy continuum

When we start any exercise the demand for energy will rise rapidly. All the energy systems contribute during all types of activity but one of them will be the predominant energy provider. The *intensity* and *duration* of the activity are the factors that decide which will be the main energy system in use. For example, jogging is a long-duration, sub-maximal exercise so the aerobic system will be the predominant energy system. An explosive, short-duration activity such as the 100 m will use the ATP-PC system. However, in a game there will be a mix of all three energy systems and the performer will move from one energy system to another. This continual movement between the thresholds of each energy system is known as the energy continuum.

Tasks to tackle 1.2

Copy and complete the table below by giving examples from a game of your choice to show when each of the three energy systems will be used.

Name of game	ATP-PC system	Lactate anaerobic system	Aerobic system

The energy continuum is often explained in terms of thresholds. The ATP-PC/lactic acid threshold is the point at which the ATP-PC energy system is exhausted and the lactate anaerobic system takes over. This is shown in Figure 1.10 at 10 seconds, with lactic acid production then peaking at 1 minute. The lactic acid/aerobic threshold, shown in Figure 1.10 at 3 minutes, is the point at which the lactate anaerobic system is exhausted and the aerobic system takes over.

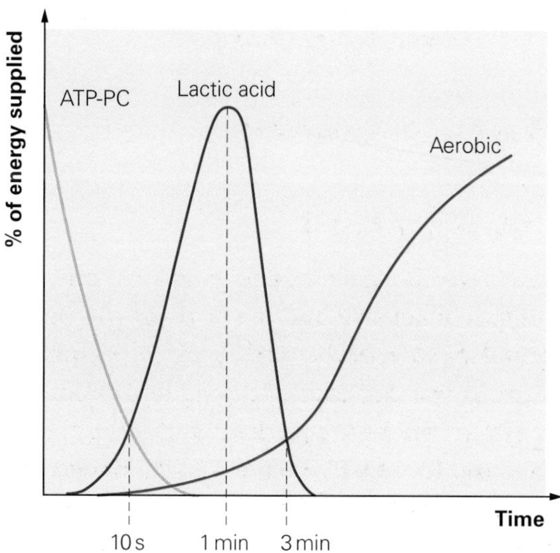

Figure 1.10 The energy continuum

Practice makes perfect

1 The marathon is an athletic event that involves performers undertaking a long-distance run over 26 miles. What would be the major energy sources used by a marathon runner? *(3 marks)*

2 In team games, players need to manage physiological demands during performance. The diagram below shows the average proportions of carbohydrate and fat usage during a period of exercise of increasing intensity.

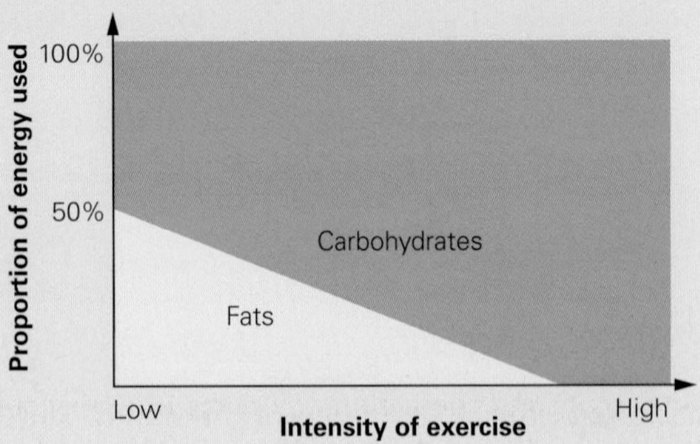

Describe what this diagram shows and explain, using your knowledge of energy systems, why this occurs. *(6 marks)*

3 Name the main energy system being used in the 100 m and explain how this system provides energy for the working muscles. *(4 marks)*

Chapter 2 Fatigue and recovery

Applied physiology to optimise performance

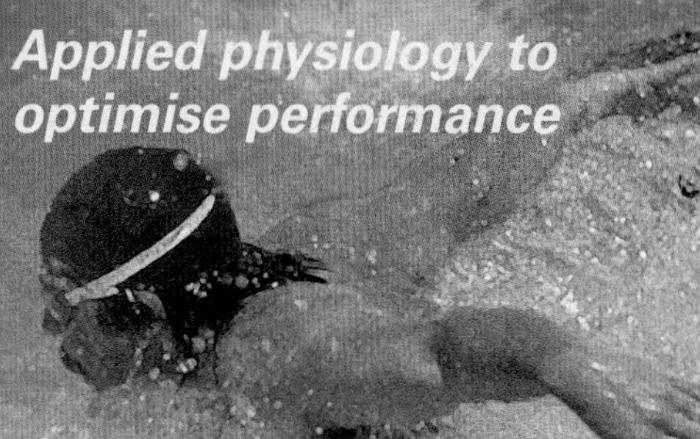

What you need to know

By the end of this chapter you should be able to:

- list the causes of fatigue
- define oxygen deficit
- define EPOC
- understand the fast and slow components of recovery

Causes of fatigue

There are many causes of fatigue and these depend on the intensity and duration of the activity. For example, a marathon runner will fatigue through glycogen depletion, whereas an 800 m runner will fatigue through lactic acid build-up.

Glycogen depletion

Glycogen stores are limited and the body has enough to last for approximately 90 minutes. When glycogen stores are depleted athletes are said to 'hit the wall' as the body tries to metabolise fat but is unable to use fat as a fuel on its own.

Lactic acid build-up

An accumulation of lactic acid releases hydrogen ions. These hydrogen ions cause an increase in the acidity of the blood plasma. This inhibits enzyme action and therefore the breakdown of glucose, and irritates nerve endings, causing pain.

Reduced rate of ATP synthesis

When stores of ATP and PC are depleted there is insufficient ATP to sustain muscular contractions.

Dehydration

Water is lost through sweating during exercise and if it is not replaced then dehydration occurs. Dehydration can have an effect on blood flow to the working muscles and result in a loss of electrolytes, such as calcium, which help with muscular contractions. Blood viscosity increases and blood pressure reduces. There is a reduction in sweating to prevent further water loss, which in turn increases core body temperature. This results in the performer being unable to meet the demands of the activity.

Reduced levels of calcium

For muscle contraction to occur there has to be a release of calcium. When there is an increase in hydrogen ions, this decreases the amount of calcium that is released from the sarcoplasmic reticulum, thus affecting muscle contraction.

Reduced levels of acetylcholine

Acetylcholine is a neurotransmitter that can help a nerve impulse to jump the synaptic cleft (the gap that separates the nerve ending from the muscle fibre) and initiate muscular contraction. When levels of acetylcholine are low, the muscles become fatigued.

Thermoregulation

During exercise, heat is generated in the body as a result of all the chemical reactions (metabolic processes) that take place to produce energy. Long-distance runners can sometimes experience difficulty with temperature regulation. The heat that is produced through muscle contraction raises the core body temperature, which causes blood viscosity to increase and metabolic processes to slow down. This means the performer is unable to sweat efficiently and dehydration occurs.

> Key term
> **Thermoregulation:** keeping body temperature maintained within certain boundaries.

TopFoto

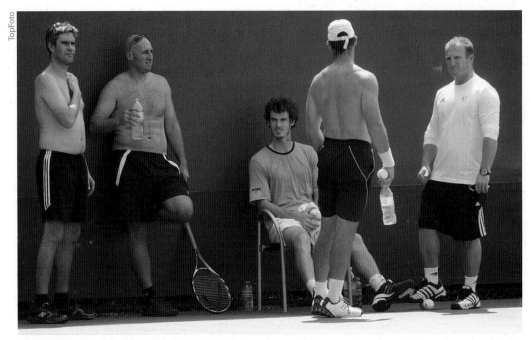

British athletes train in camps in other countries to prepare for hot weather competitions

The thermoregulatory centre in the medulla oblongata controls temperature. Heat is transported to the surface of the skin by the blood and the blood vessels vasodilate, enabling heat to be lost through radiation, convection or through the evaporation of sweat.

When the body is dehydrated, total blood volume decreases. More blood is redirected to the skin (to aid cooling), so the amount of blood and therefore oxygen available to the working muscles is reduced and this affects performance. In hot conditions this situation is exacerbated, so it is important to acclimatise, enabling the body to modify the control systems that regulate blood flow to the skin and sweating.

Offsetting fatigue

There are ways to limit the onset of fatigue and to reduce its impact:

- The relevant energy system can be trained using an appropriate training method. For example, continuous training uses the aerobic system.
- Glycogen levels can be conserved by pacing activity levels. Marathon runners, for example, pace themselves, as going too fast early in the race will speed up glycogen metabolism.
- Glycogen levels can be increased before an event to enable an endurance-based activity to last for longer. This is known as glycogen loading (see Chapter 5).
- Blood glucose levels can be boosted by keeping hydrated. Athletes should drink fluid with a carbohydrate level of no more than 6% throughout a performance.

The recovery process

The recovery process involves returning the body to the state it was in before exercise. The reactions that occur and how long the process takes depend on the duration and intensity of the exercise undertaken and the individual's level of fitness. During recovery, heart and breathing rates remain high in order to continue taking in large amounts of oxygen. This oxygen is then used to return the body to its pre-exercise state.

Tasks to tackle 2.1

Copy and complete the table below to show the changes that take place during exercise.

Factor	Change
Temperature	
ATP stores	
Phosphocreatine stores	
Glycogen stores	
Triglyceride stores	
Carbon dioxide levels	
Oxygen/myoglobin stores	
Lactic acid levels	

Excess post-exercise oxygen consumption (EPOC)

After strenuous exercise there are four main tasks that need to be completed before the exhausted muscle can operate at full efficiency again:

- replacement of ATP and phosphocreatine (the fast replenishment stage)
- replenishment of myoglobin with oxygen
- removal of lactic acid (the slow replenishment stage)
- replacement of glycogen

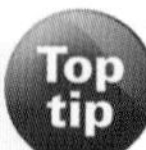

Top tip Questions in the exam often ask about the importance of taking in extra oxygen.

Key term **EPOC (excess post-exercise oxygen consumption):** the process by which more oxygen is consumed during recovery from exercise than would have been consumed at rest during the same time.

Figure 2.1 The processes involved in EPOC

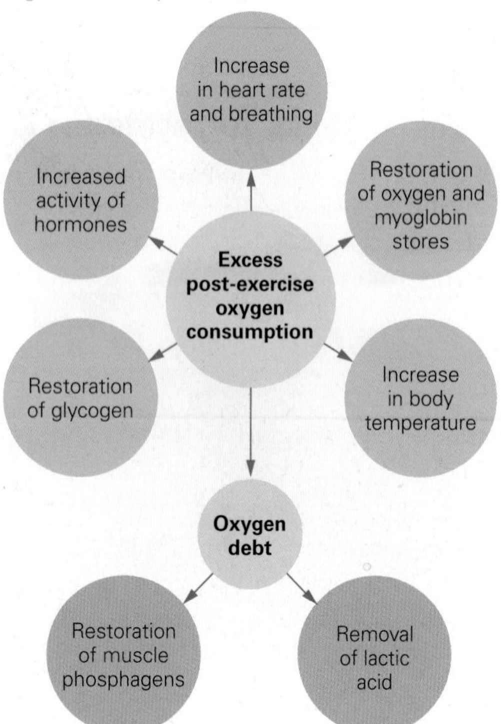

The first three of these tasks require a large amount of oxygen. Therefore, during recovery the body takes in elevated amounts of oxygen and transports it to the working muscles to maintain elevated rates of aerobic respiration. This surplus energy is then used to help return the body to its pre-exercise state. This process is known as **excess post-exercise oxygen consumption (EPOC).**

The processes that take place during EPOC are summarised in Figure 2.1.

When we start to exercise, insufficient oxygen is distributed to the tissues for all the energy production to be met aerobically, so the two anaerobic systems have to be used. The amount of oxygen that the subject was short of during the exercise is known as the **oxygen deficit**. This is compensated for by the surplus amount of oxygen — or **oxygen debt** — that results from EPOC. However, oxygen debt does not always equal oxygen deficit because oxygen is used during recovery to provide energy to maintain elevated heart and breathing rates.

Let's look at the four tasks involved in EPOC in more detail.

The fast replenishment stage

During the fast replenishment stage (also known as the **alactacid component**), elevated rates of respiration continue to supply oxygen to provide the energy

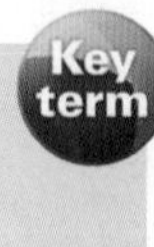

Key term **Fast replenishment:** the restoration of ATP and phosphocreatine stores and the re-saturation of myoglobin with oxygen.

for ATP production and phosphocreatine replenishment. Complete restoration of phosphocreatine takes up to 3 minutes, but 50% of stores can be replenished after only 30 seconds, during which time approximately 3 litres of oxygen are consumed. Figure 2.2 shows the relationship between recovery time and the replenishment of muscle phosphagens (ATP and phosphocreatine) after exercise.

This knowledge is useful for a coach or performer who will want to prevent the use of the lactate anaerobic system with its fatiguing by-product. A time-out in basketball will allow for significant restoration of PC stores.

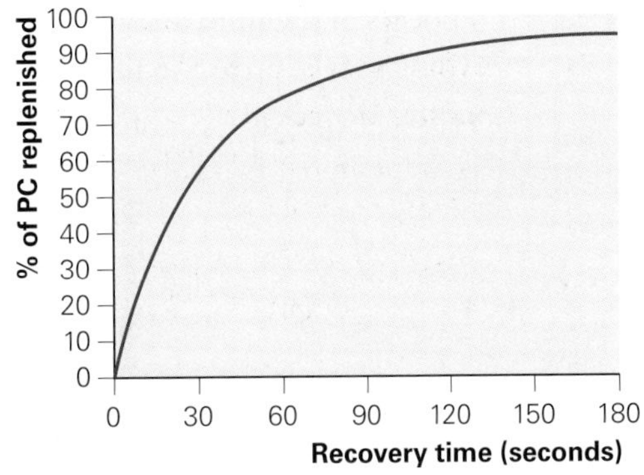

Figure 2.2 Recovery time and PC regeneration

Tasks to tackle 2.2

In most team games it is possible to create a 30-second rest to replenish PC stores. Think of three instances when you could employ these tactics.

1 ....

2 ....

3 ....

Myoglobin and replenishment of oxygen stores

Myoglobin has a high affinity for oxygen. It stores oxygen in the muscle and transports it from the capillaries to the mitochondria for energy provision. After exercise, oxygen stores in the myoglobin are limited. The surplus of oxygen supplied through EPOC helps replenish these stores, taking up to 2 minutes and using approximately 0.5 litres of oxygen.

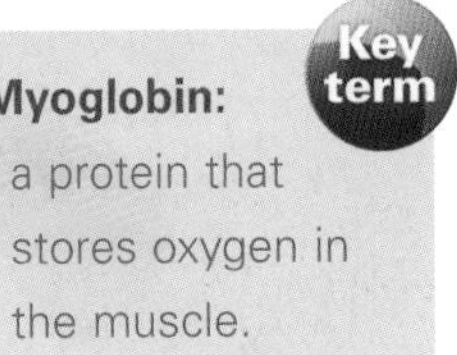

Myoglobin: a protein that stores oxygen in the muscle.

The slow replenishment stage

This stage is concerned with the removal of lactic acid and is also known as the **lactacid component**. It is the slower of the two replenishment processes and full recovery may take up to an hour, depending on the intensity and duration of the exercise. Lactic acid can be removed in four ways, as shown in Table 2.1.

The majority of lactic acid can be oxidised, so performing a cool-down accelerates its removal because exercise keeps the metabolic rate of muscles high and keeps capillaries dilated. This means that oxygen can be flushed through, removing the accumulated lactic acid. The lactacid oxygen recovery begins as soon as lactic acid

Table 2.1 Component stages of lactic acid removal

Destination	Approximate % lactic acid involved
Oxidation into carbon dioxide and water in the inactive muscles and organs	65
Conversion into glycogen — then stored in muscles/liver	20
Conversion into protein	10
Conversion into glucose	5

appears in the muscle cell and continues, using breathed oxygen, until recovery is complete. This can take up to 5–6 litres of oxygen in the first half hour of recovery, removing up to 50% of the lactic acid.

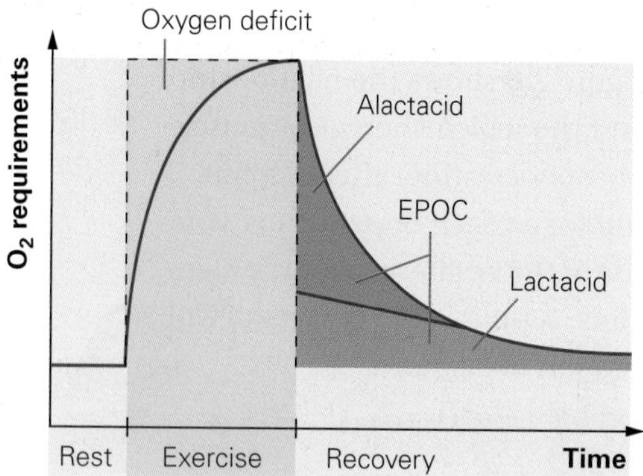

Figure 2.3 Recovery after maximal exercise

Glycogen replenishment

Glycogen, as the main fuel for the aerobic system and lactate anaerobic system, is depleted during exercise. The stores of glycogen in relation to the stores of fat are relatively small, so it is important to conserve glycogen in order not to cross the lactate threshold. The replacement of glycogen stores depends on the type of exercise undertaken, and when and how much carbohydrate is consumed following exercise. It may take several days to complete the restoration of glycogen after a marathon, but a significant amount of glycogen can be restored in less than an hour after long-duration, low-intensity exercise. Eating a high-carbohydrate meal will accelerate glycogen restoration, as will eating within 1 hour following exercise.

Factors affecting recovery

Increase in breathing and heart rates

This is important to assist in recovery as extra oxygen is required to return the body to its pre-exercise state. However, the increase in breathing and heart rates requires additional extra oxygen to provide energy for the muscles of the heart and respiratory system.

Increased activity of hormones

The continuation of sub-maximal exercise (such as a cool-down) will keep hormone levels elevated and this will keep respiratory and metabolic levels high so that extra oxygen can be taken in.

Top tip

Questions on EPOC often involve a description of the fast and slow replenishment stages.

Increase in body temperature

When temperature remains high, respiratory rates will also remain high and this will help the performer take in more oxygen during recovery. However, extra oxygen is needed to fuel this increase in temperature until the body returns to normal.

Practice makes perfect

1 At the end of an 800 m swim, the swimmer will be out of breath and will continue to breathe heavily even though he/she has come to a complete rest. Explain why this breathlessness occurs. *(4 marks)*

2 State what the letters A and B represent on the graph below. *(2 marks)*

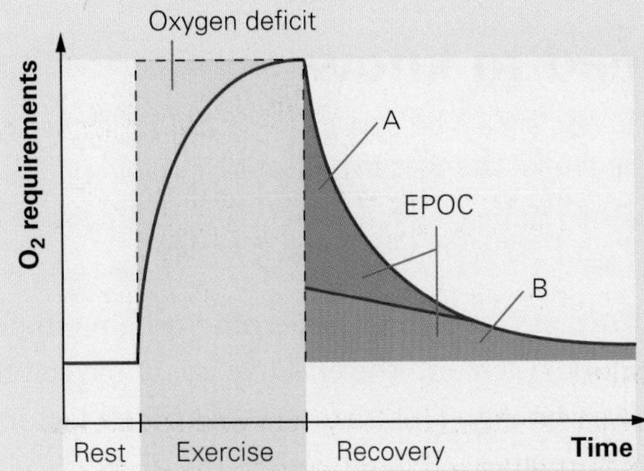

3 Explain how lactic acid is removed from the blood by the body. *(4 marks)*

Chapter 3

Applied physiology to optimise performance

What makes a successful endurance performance?

What you need to know

By the end of this chapter you should be able to:

- define VO_2 max and list the factors that can affect it
- define OBLA and list its effects
- understand the relationship between OBLA and VO_2 max

A good endurance performer can utilise the aerobic system efficiently through both the effective transportation of oxygen and the effective use of oxygen to break down glycogen, fats and proteins to release energy. This chapter looks at the factors that can contribute to successful endurance performance.

Significance of maximum oxygen consumption in sporting performance

VO_2 max is the maximum volume of oxygen that can be taken in and used by the muscles per minute. A person's VO_2 max will determine endurance performance in sport. Average VO_2 max for an A-level student is around 45–55 ml kg^{-1} min^{-1} for males and 35–44 ml kg^{-1} min^{-1} for females.

VO_2 max depends on:

- how effectively an individual can inspire and expire
- once he/she has inspired, how effective the transportation of the oxygen is from the lungs to where it is needed
- how well that oxygen is then used

> **Key term**
>
> **VO_2 max:** the maximum volume of oxygen that can be taken in and used by the muscles per minute.

Factors affecting VO_2 max

VO_2 max is affected by a number of factors:

Lifestyle

Smoking, a sedentary lifestyle and poor diet can all reduce VO_2 max values.

Training

VO_2 max can be improved by up to 10–20% following a period of aerobic training (continuous, fartlek and aerobic interval).

Body composition

Research has shown that VO_2 max decreases as the percentage of body fat increases.

Differences in gender

A male endurance athlete will have a VO_2 max of around 70 ml kg^{-1} min^{-1}, whereas a female endurance athlete will have a VO_2 max of around 60 ml kg^{-1} min^{-1}. This is because the average female is smaller than the average male. Females have:

- a smaller left ventricle and therefore a lower stroke volume
- a lower maximum cardiac output
- a lower blood volume, which results in a lower haemoglobin level
- lower tidal and ventilatory volumes

TopFoto

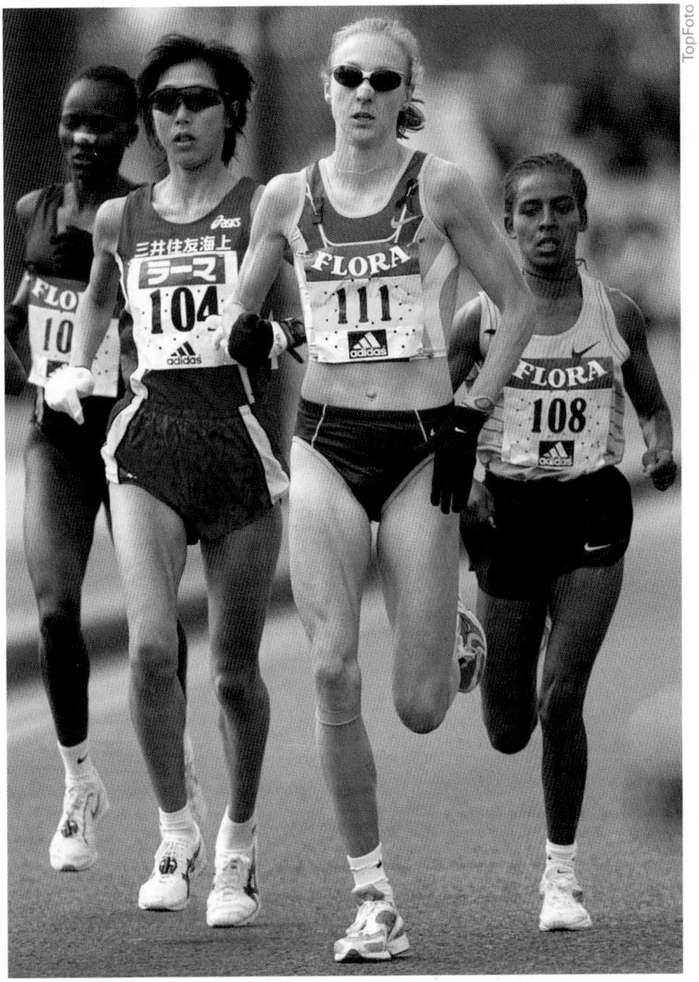

Paula Radcliffe's VO_2 max is around 80 ml kg^{-1} min^{-1}. This means she has more oxygen going to the muscles and can use this oxygen to provide energy to enable a high rate of exercise.

Differences in age

As we get older our VO_2 max declines as our body systems become less efficient:

- Maximum heart rate drops by around 5–7 beats per minute per decade.
- An increase in peripheral resistance results in a decrease of maximal stroke volume.
- Blood pressure increases both at rest and during exercise.
- Less air is exchanged in the lungs due to a decline in vital capacity and an increase in residual air.

Physiological adaptations

Regular aerobic exercise increases VO_2 max due to the following physiological changes that take place:

- increased maximum cardiac output
- increased stroke volume/ejection fraction/cardiac hypertrophy
- greater heart rate range

- less oxygen being used for heart muscle, so more available to muscles
- increased arterio-venous oxygen difference (A-VO_2 diff) — the difference in oxygen content between the arteries and the veins
- increased blood volume and haemoglobin/red blood cells/blood count
- increased stores of glycogen and triglycerides
- increased myoglobin (content of muscle)
- increased capillarisation (of muscle)
- increased number and size of mitochondria
- increased concentrations of oxidative enzymes
- increased lactate tolerance
- reduced body fat
- slow twitch hypertrophy

Evaluation of VO_2 max

There are various methods of evaluating VO_2 max.

The **Douglas bag** is an accurate method carried out under laboratory conditions. The athlete runs on a treadmill, to the point of exhaustion — i.e. it is a maximal text. The air that is expired is collected in a Douglas bag. The concentration of oxygen in the expired air is then measured and compared with the percentage of oxygen that is in atmospheric air to see how much oxygen has been used during the task. This test requires access to expensive hi-tech equipment, so less expensive predictive tests (indirect tests) have been developed to estimate the performer's VO_2 max.

One such test is the **multistage fitness test** developed by the National Coaching Foundation. The athlete performs a 20 m progressive shuttle run in time with a bleep, to the point of exhaustion. The level reached depends on the number of shuttle runs completed and is ascertained from a standard results table.

This test gives only an estimate of VO_2 max and is nowhere near as accurate as the Douglas bag test. However, it does provide a guide from which progress can be monitored, and is easy to set up. The equipment required is limited, making it a cheap alternative. It is also possible to test large numbers of people simultaneously, so it is not as time consuming as the Douglas bag test.

The **Harvard step test** involves the athlete stepping up and down rhythmically on a bench for 5 minutes. The recovery heart rate is then measured and used to predict VO_2 max. The **PWC170 cycle ergometer test** involves three consecutive 4-minute workloads on a cycle ergometer. The heart rate for each workload is plotted on a graph and a line of best fit is drawn. Both this test and the Harvard step test are sub-maximal. The **Cooper 12-minute run** requires the athlete to run as far as he/she can in 12 minutes and the distance covered is recorded and compared to a standardised table. In this test the performer runs to exhaustion.

Onset of blood lactate accumulation (OBLA)

Lactate is produced when hydrogen is removed from the lactic acid molecule. **Onset of blood lactate accumulation** (**OBLA**) is the point at which lactate starts to accumulate in the blood. At rest, approximately 1–2 millimoles per litre (mmol l^{-1}) of lactic acid can be found in the blood. However, during intense exercise, levels of lactic acid rise dramatically. Lactate levels in the blood start to accumulate when the concentration of lactic acid is around 4 mmol l^{-1}.

Measuring OBLA gives an indication of endurance capacity. Some individuals can work at higher levels of intensity than others before OBLA and can delay when the threshold occurs. OBLA is expressed as a percentage of VO_2 max. An average untrained individual will work at approximately 50–60% of VO_2 max, whereas a trained endurance performer can work at around 85–90% of VO_2 max before OBLA occurs.

> **Key term**
>
> **Onset of blood lactate accumulation (OBLA):** the point at which lactate starts to accumulate in the blood.

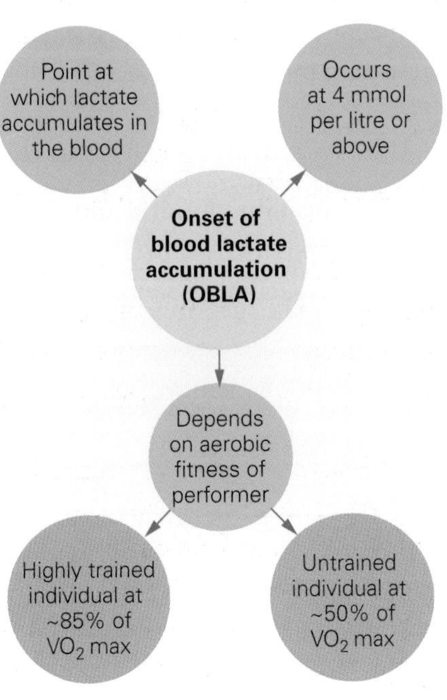

Figure 3.1 Summary of OBLA

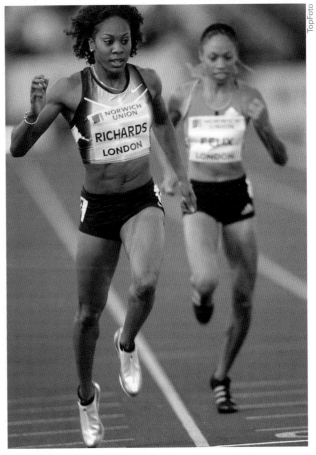

Runners finish a 400m race with a blood lactate concentration that is 20–25 times higher than resting level

TopFoto

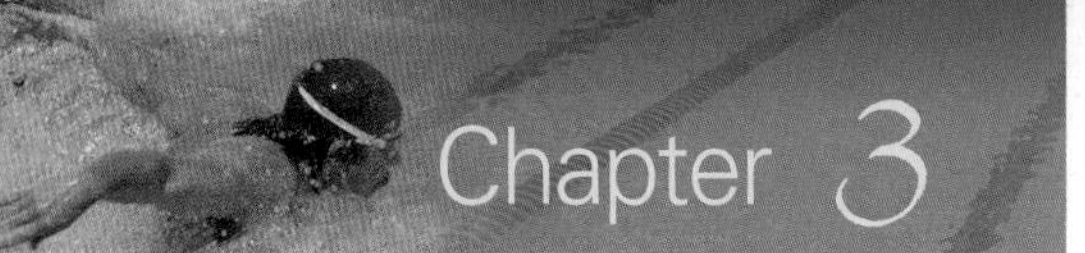

Buffering is a process that aids the removal of lactic acid and maintains acidity levels in the blood and muscle. A trained performer can cope with higher levels of blood lactate and can speed up its removal.

The multistage fitness test is a good example to illustrate OBLA. The performer reaches a point, due to the increasing intensity of this test, where energy cannot be provided aerobically. This means that the performer has to use the anaerobic systems to regenerate ATP. Blood lactate levels start to increase until eventually muscle fatigue occurs and the performer slows down and is no longer able to keep up with the bleep.

Factors affecting the rate of lactate accumulation

Exercise intensity

The higher the exercise intensity, the greater the demand for energy (ATP). Fast twitch fibres are used for high-intensity exercise and can only maintain their workload with the use of glycogen as a fuel. When glycogen is broken down in the absence of oxygen into pyruvic acid, lactic acid is formed.

Muscle fibre type

Slow twitch fibres produce less lactate than fast twitch fibres. When slow twitch fibres use glycogen as a fuel, due to the presence of oxygen, the glycogen can be broken down much more effectively and with little lactate production.

Rate of blood lactate removal

If the rate of lactate removal is equivalent to the rate of lactate production then the concentration of blood lactate remains constant. If lactate production increases then lactate will start to accumulate in the blood until OBLA is reached.

Training

Adaptations occur to trained muscles. Increased numbers of mitochondria and levels of myoglobin, together with an increase in capillary density, improve the capacity for aerobic respiration and therefore help to reduce the use of the lactate anaerobic system.

Practice makes perfect

1 It is important as a games player to have a good VO_2 max. What is meant by the term VO_2 max? *(2 marks)*

2 Suggest five structural and/or physiological causes of the difference in VO_2 max between a trained and an untrained performer. *(5 marks)*

3 Describe and explain how lactate threshold varies as fitness improves. *(3 marks)*

Chapter 4

Applied physiology to optimise performance

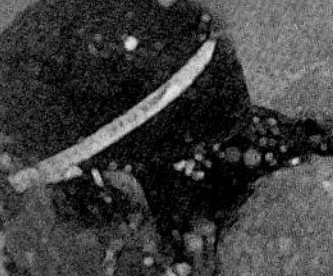

Structure and function of muscles

What you need to know

By the end of this chapter you should be able to:

- identify the structure and function of muscle
- list the characteristics of the three fibre types: slow twitch (type I), fast oxidative glycolytic (type IIa) and fast glycolytic (type IIb)
- understand the sliding filament hypothesis, including the structure of actin and myosin, the chemicals required to create movement and the process that occurs to create movement
- understand motor units and recruitment
- understand muscle innervation

This chapter looks at the structure and function of skeletal muscle and how knowledge of this can impact on and improve performance.

Skeletal muscle is often referred to as voluntary, striped or striated muscle due to its appearance (see Figure 4.1). Skeletal muscle is surrounded by a layer of connective tissue called the epimysium. This consists mainly of collagen fibres and its function is to provide a smooth surface for other muscles to glide against. Skeletal muscle is made up of bundles of muscle fibres, which are enclosed in a connective tissue sheath called the perimysium. Each of the individual muscle fibres is made up of many smaller fibres called myofibrils. Myofibrils are covered by a thin layer of connective tissue or endomysium.

The epimysium, perimysium and endomysium are all connected to one another so that when the muscle fibres contract, movement occurs through their links with the tendons and their attachment to bones at joints.

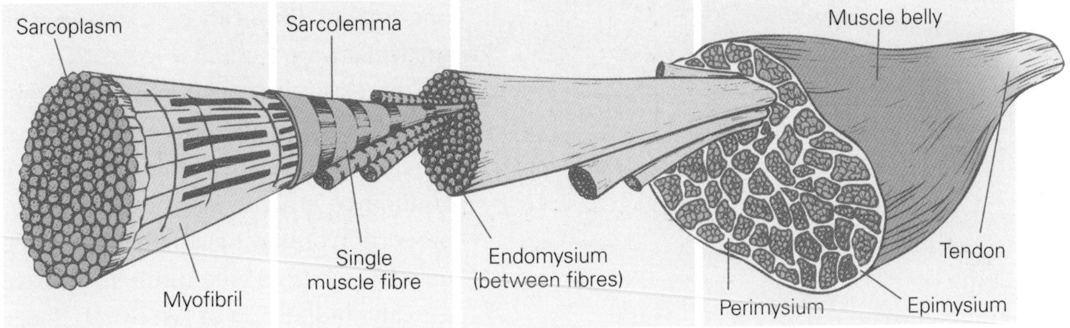

Figure 4.1 The structure of skeletal muscle

Control of muscular contraction

Muscle action has to be controlled in order for movement to be effective. There are several internal regulatory mechanisms that make this possible.

Proprioceptors

These are sense organs in the muscles, tendons and joints that inform the body of the extent of movement that has taken place.

Muscle spindle apparatus

These are very sensitive proprioceptors that lie between skeletal muscle fibres. They provide information about the changes in muscle length and the rate of change in muscle length. When the muscle stretches, the spindle also stretches and this sends an impulse to the spinal cord. If the muscle is stretched too far, the muscle spindle apparatus alters tension within the muscle, causing a stretch reflex, which automatically shortens the muscle.

Golgi tendon organs

These are thin pockets of connective tissue that occur where the muscle fibre and tendon meet. They provide information to the central nervous system concerning the degree of tension or stretch within the muscle. When stretched, they trigger both the reflex inhibition of the muscle that is contracting and stretching the tendon, as well as the reflex contraction of the antagonist muscle.

Types of muscle fibre

Three main types of muscle fibre can be identified, namely type I (slow oxidative), type IIa (fast oxidative glycolytic) and type IIb (fast glycolytic). Our skeletal muscles contain a mixture of all three types of fibre but not in equal proportions. The mix is mainly genetically determined. These fibres are grouped into motor units where only one type of fibre can be found in one particular unit.

Table 4.1 The characteristics of muscle fibre types

Characteristic	Type I	Type IIa	Type IIb
Contraction speed ($m\,s^{-1}$)	slow (110)	fast (50)	fast (50)
Motor neurone size	small	large	large
Force produced	low	high	high
Fatiguability	low	medium	high
Mitochondrial density	high	medium	low
Myoglobin content	high	medium	low
Glycogen store	low	high	high
Triglyceride store	high	medium	low
Capillary density	high	medium	low
Aerobic capacity	high	medium	low
Anaerobic capacity	low	medium	high

The relative proportion of each fibre type varies in the same muscles of different people. For example, an elite endurance athlete will have a greater proportion of slow twitch fibres in the leg muscles, while an elite sprinter will have a greater proportion of fast twitch fibres. Postural muscles tend to have a greater proportion of slow twitch fibres as they are involved in maintaining body position over long periods of time.

All three fibre types have specific characteristics, as shown in Table 4.1, that allow them to perform their role successfully.

Top tip
Questions are frequently asked on the characteristics of the fibre types, so learn them!

The effect of training on fibre type

Fibre type appears to be genetically determined. However, it is possible to increase the size of muscle fibres through training. This increase in size (hypertrophy) is caused by an increase in the number and size of myofibrils per fibre, with a consequent increase in the amount of proteins, namely myosin. As a result, there will be greater strength in the muscle.

Tasks to tackle 4.1

Copy the table below and think of three sporting examples for each category.

Slow twitch (type I)	Fast twitch (type IIa)	Fast twitch (type IIb)
(1)	(1)	(1)
(2)	(2)	(2)
(3)	(3)	(3)

The sliding filament hypothesis

In order to understand how a muscle contracts it is important to look at the detailed structure of a myofibril. This is the contractile unit of the muscle that runs the length of the fibre.

Under a microscope it is possible to see cross-bands or striations running across the myofibril. This pattern of cross-banding is repeated along the length of the myofibril. The repeated unit is called a sarcomere. Each sarcomere contains two types of protein filament: the thick myosin filaments and the thin actin filaments. During contraction, these two slide across one another and connect or make cross-bridges. This overlapping creates the striped appearance of the sarcomere (see Figure 4.1 on page 23).

A sarcomere is constructed in the following way:

- Z lines are at the borders of the sarcomere
- I bands are the areas near the edge of the sarcomere containing only actin filaments
- A bands are the regions where actin and myosin overlap and correspond to the length of the myosin filaments
- H zones are areas in the centre of the A bands containing only myosin

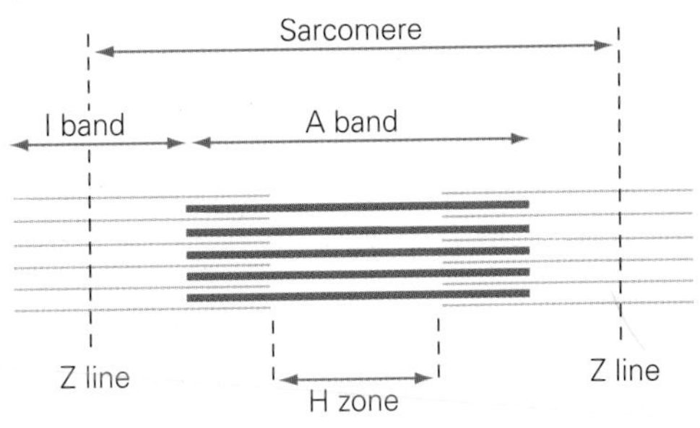

Figure 4.2 The structure of a sarcomere

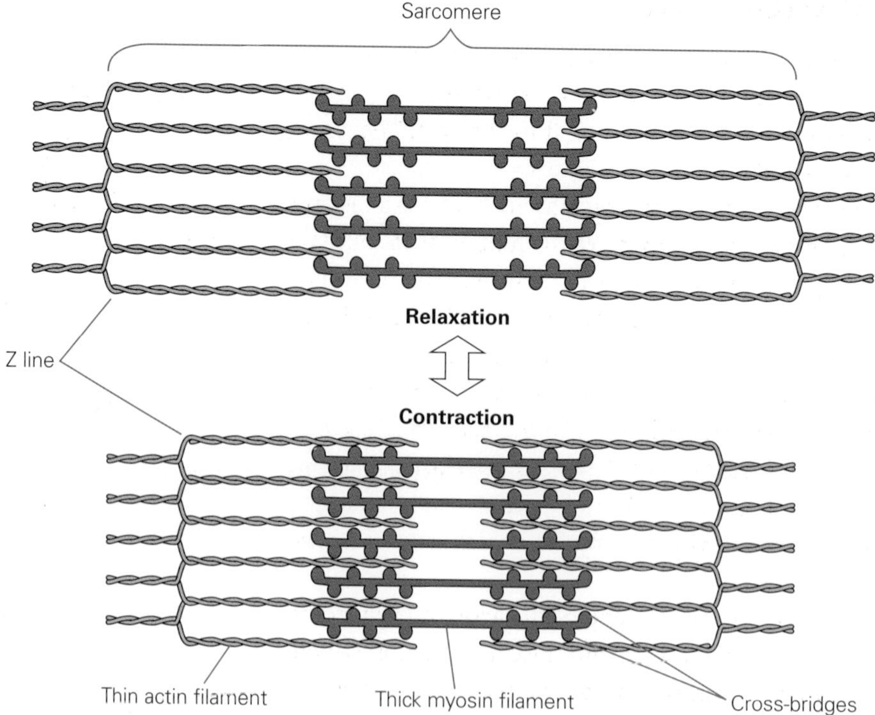

Figure 4.3 The sliding filament theory of muscle contraction

The actin has binding sites and the myosin can attach to these through tiny protein projections that look similar to a golf club in appearance. Each of these projections contains ATP-ase, the enzyme used to break down ATP, which provides the energy to bind the myosin cross-bridge onto the actin filament and allow muscular contraction to take place (see Figure 4.3).

As a muscle contracts:

- the Z lines come closer together
- the width of the I bands decreases
- the width of the H zones decreases
- there is no change in the width of the A band

The actin filament also contains two molecules called troponin and tropomyosin. These cover the binding sites of the actin and prevent cross-bridges from forming. This can be overcome by the release of calcium from the sarcoplasmic reticulum, which attracts the troponin, neutralises the tropomyosin and releases the binding sites on the actin, allowing cross-bridges to occur.

This sliding filament hypothesis works rather like a ratchet mechanism where the cross-bridges constantly attach, detach then reattach with the net result of shortening the sarcomere.

The motor unit

Muscle innervation occurs when an impulse travels from the cerebrum or spinal cord. These impulses travel along nerves (neurones) to the muscle and cause it to contract. The structure of a nerve cell is shown in Figure 4.4.

The dendrites receive impulses from other neurones and pass them on to the cell body. The cell body sorts out the information and sends an impulse down the axon, or motor neurone. These impulses are electrical impulses, similar to electric currents in a wire. To protect them, an insulator called the myelin sheath, made up of fatty material, surrounds the axon. The myelin sheath is absent at intervals along the axon. These breaks are called nodes of Ranvier. The impulse travels from one node of Ranvier to the next, which results in it travelling quicker. The thicker the myelin sheath, the faster the impulse is conducted.

As the impulse reaches the end of the axon, it triggers the release of acetycholine at the neuromuscular junction (where the axon connects with the motor end plate of the muscle).

One motor neurone cannot stimulate the whole muscle. Instead, a motor neurone will stimulate a number of fibres (between 15 and 2000) within that muscle. This whole system — one motor neurone and its corresponding muscle fibres — is called a motor unit. Each motor unit contains only one kind of muscle fibre, for example only slow oxidative fibres.

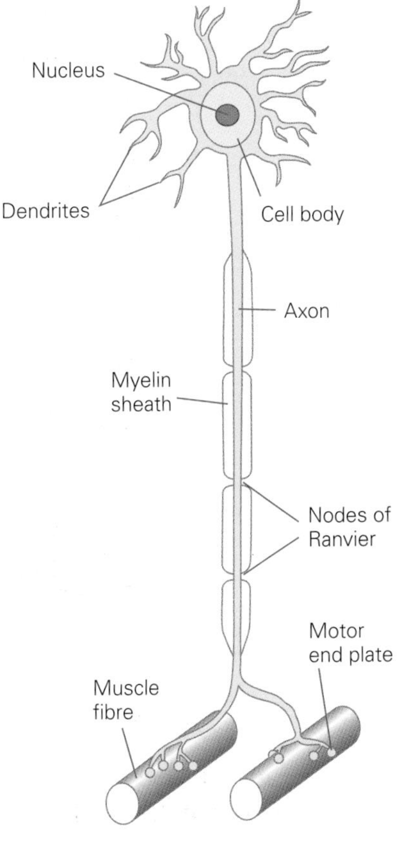

Figure 4.4 A nerve cell

Characteristics of the motor unit

The all-or-none law

A minimum amount of stimulation, called the threshold, is required to start a muscle contraction. If an impulse is equal to or more than the threshold then all the muscle fibres in a motor unit will contract. However, if the impulse is less than the threshold then no muscle action will occur. As such, the motor unit exhibits an all-or-none response.

Gradation of contraction

This refers to the strength or force exerted by a muscle and is dependent on the following:

- **Recruitment** — the greater the number of motor units that are recruited, the greater the number of muscle fibres that will contract, therefore increasing the force that can be produced. This can also be referred to as **multiple unit summation**.
- **Frequency** — the greater the frequency of stimuli, the greater the tension developed by the muscle. If the stimuli occur very infrequently, the calcium concentration in the sarcomere

returns to resting levels before the arrival of the next stimulus (Figure 4.5a). When the stimuli occur frequently, not all the calcium released in response to the first stimulus is taken back into the sarcoplasmic reticulum. As a result, summation occurs (Figure 4.5b). This is also called **wave summation** (where summation means the addition of motor units), where repeated activation of a motor neurone stimulating a given muscle fibre results in summation.

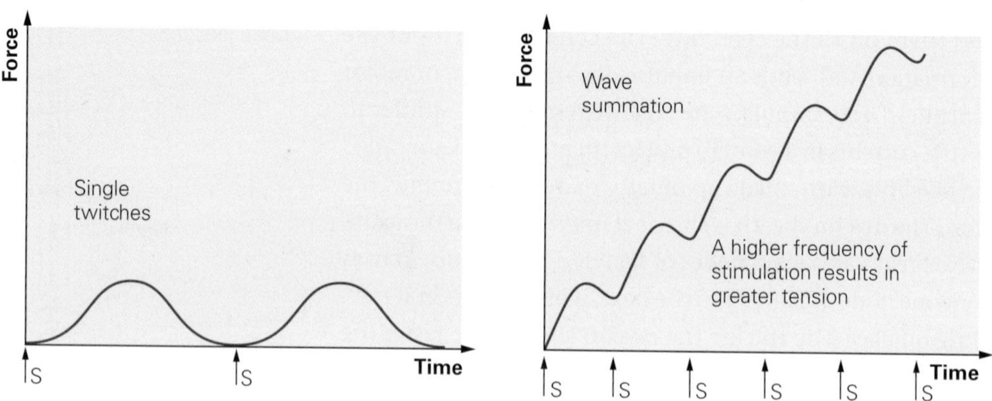

Figure 4.5 (a) Low-frequency stimuli; (b) high-frequency stimuli leading to increased tension

- **Timing** — If all the motor units are stimulated at exactly the same time, then maximum force can be applied. This is referred to as **spatial summation** or **synchronisation**.

Practice makes perfect

1 When jumping up for a rebound in basketball, players rely on their muscles to produce maximal contractions. What are the characteristics of the type of muscle fibres used to produce these maximal contractions? *(6 marks)*

2 Identify four structural and/or physiological differences between fast and slow twitch muscle fibres. *(4 marks)*

3 Weightlifting is a sport where the performer generates maximal strength contractions. Explain what you understand by the term motor unit and describe how motor units can be used to produce muscle contractions of varying strength. *(5 marks)*

Chapter 5

Applied physiology to optimise performance

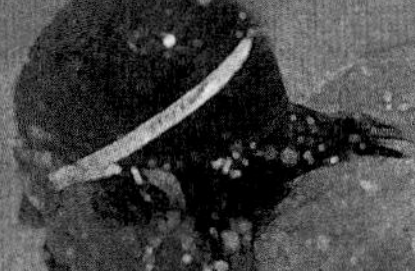

Sports supplements

What you need to know

By the end of this chapter you should be able to:

- list supplements and ergogenic aids and explain what they are, discuss the advantages and disadvantages of their use and identify which athletes use them
- understand how to prepare the body for training and performance through water and electrolyte balance, achieving optimal weight and diet
- say how this is achieved for different performers, for example endurance athlete versus power athlete

Sports supplements

Supplements are often used to increase energy stores, which in turn enhance athletic performance. A supplement is something that can be added to the diet, typically to make up for a nutritional deficiency.

Creatine monohydrate

Creatine monohydrate is a supplement used to increase the amount of phosphocreatine stored in the muscles. It allows the ATP-PC system to operate for longer and can help to improve recovery times. Athletes in explosive events such as sprints, jumps and throws are likely to experience the most benefits. Possible side effects include dehydration, bloating, muscle cramps and slight liver damage. Studies suggest, however, that a daily intake of 5 grams or over usually ends up in the urine rather than in the muscle.

Herbal remedies

Herbal remedies are often advertised as 'natural' products that have effects ranging from decreasing body fat to elevating blood testosterone levels, increasing muscle mass, enhancing energy, improving strength and stamina, and generally improving health and athletic performance. However, many of these claims are unfounded and care should be taken by athletes who use them. A simple internet search shows herbal remedies in their thousands: electrolyte stamina tablets for athletes who experience a lot of fluid loss, whey protein powder to increase muscle metabolism, 'gotu kola' powder to enhance mental alertness, and so on. More common remedies include ginseng, which is used to increase endurance and enhance muscle recovery.

Protein supplements

Athletes may use protein supplements to enhance muscle repair and growth. This can result in better endurance and increase muscle strength and size. Protein supplements are usually taken by strength athletes who believe that protein is important to build muscle as well as repair and rebuild muscle that is broken down during strenuous exercise. However, a diet high in protein can put a strain on the liver and kidneys and can cause a negative nitrogen balance, which slows down muscle growth and can cause fatigue.

Sodium bicarbonate

The concept behind drinking a solution of sodium bicarbonate is that it reduces the acidity in the muscle cells. This delays fatigue and allows the performer to continue exercising at high intensity for longer. Sodium bicarbonate increases the buffering capacity of the blood, so it can neutralise the negative effects of lactic acid. However, it can also result in vomiting, pain, cramping, diarrhoea or a feeling of being bloated. Athletes who use the lactate anaerobic system in their events, such as 400 m runners, rowers, and 100–400 m swimmers, produce a lot of acidity and will therefore benefit from 'soda loading'.

Caffeine

Caffeine is a stimulant, so it can increase mental alertness and reduce fatigue. It is also thought to improve the mobilisation of fatty acids in the body, thereby sparing muscle glycogen stores. It is taken as a supplement by endurance performers who predominantly use the aerobic system, because fats are the preferred fuel for low-intensity, long-duration exercise. The drawbacks of caffeine are the increased risk of dehydration (it is a diuretic), irritability, insomnia and anxiety.

Glycogen loading

Glycogen loading is a form of dietary manipulation involving maximising glycogen stores. It is often used by long-distance runners and is popularly known as carbo-loading. Before an important competition, a performer eats a diet high in protein and fats for 3 days and exercises at relatively high intensity so that glycogen stores are depleted.

Key term

Glycogen loading: a dietary strategy to maximise the storage of glycogen in the muscles.

Table 5.1 The advantages and disadvantages of glycogen loading

Advantages of glycogen loading	Disadvantages of glycogen loading
Increased glycogen synthesis Increased glycogen stores in the muscle Delays fatigue Increases endurance capacity	Water retention, which results in bloating Heavy legs Affects digestion Weight increase Irritability during the depletion phase Alters the training programme

This is followed by 3 days of a diet high in carbohydrates and some very light training. Studies show that this will greatly increase the stores of glycogen in the muscle and can prevent a performer from 'hitting the wall'.

Ergogenic aids

All athletes want to improve their performance and there are both legal and illegal methods, in addition to training, for achieving this. Substances that improve performance are referred to as ergogenic aids. Table 5.2 lists some illegal ergogenic aids that, unfortunately, some athletes feel the need to use.

Top tip
Make sure you know which type of performer uses which type of aid.

Table 5.2 Uses and side effects of illegal ergogenic aids

Method of enhancement	Description	Reasons for use (benefits)	Which athletes might use them?	Side effects
Anabolic steroids	Artificially produced hormones	Promote muscle growth, strength and lean body weight	Power athletes, such as sprinters	Liver damage Heart and immune system problems Acne Behaviour changes, such as aggression, paranoia and mood swings
Human growth hormone (HGH)	Artificially produced hormone	Increases muscle mass and causes a decrease in fat	Used across a range of sports from sprinting to explosive activities such as rugby, and even to enhance endurance performance; it is not known how widespread the use of this drug is as it is difficult to detect	Heart and nerve diseases Glucose intolerance High levels of blood fats
Beta blockers	Drugs that inhibit certain autonomous nerve activity	Help to calm an individual down and decrease anxiety Can improve accuracy in precision sports through steadying the nerves	Snooker players, golfers (the PGA announced in 2007 that it would be testing its members for the use of beta blockers; it then controversially withdrew this in the 2008 British Open)	Tiredness due to low blood pressure and slower heart rate, which affect aerobic capacity
Erythropoietin (EPO)	A natural hormone produced by the kidneys to increase red blood cells; it can now be artificially manufactured	An increase in haemoglobin means an increase in the oxygen-carrying capacity of the body, which can lead to an increase in the amount of work performed	Tends to be used by endurance performers, such as Tour de France cyclists, who need effective oxygen transport	Can result in blood clotting, stroke and, in a few cases, death

Tasks to tackle 5.1

Below are pictures of an endurance performer and a power athlete. Copy and complete the boxes to show which supplements and ergogenic aids are best for that type of performer.

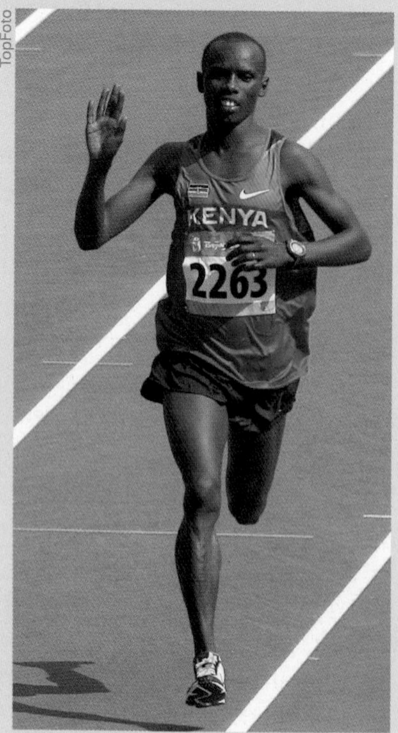

TopFoto

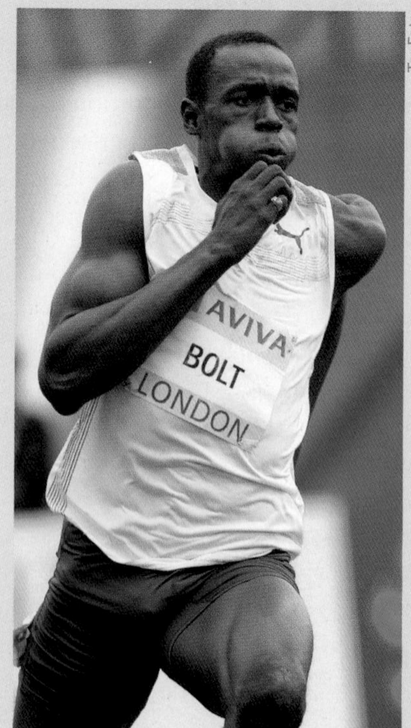

TopFoto

Supplements	
Endurance athlete	Power athlete

Ergogenic aids	
Endurance athlete	Power athlete

Preparing the body for training and performance

Water and electrolyte balance

Water is extremely important in the human body. It transports nutrients, hormones and waste products around the body. It is the main component of many cells and plays an important part in regulating body temperature.

During exercise, energy is required and some of that energy is released as heat. Sweating prevents the athlete from overheating. However, this cooling process means that water is lost from the body. Once the body starts to lose water during exercise, a decrease in blood volume can result. When this occurs, the heart has to work harder to move blood around the body and less oxygen is available to the working muscles, which in turn affects performance. It is therefore important when exercising to drink early and often.

Electrolytes are substances that become ions in solution and ions have the capacity to conduct electricity. The balance of the electrolytes in our bodies is important for the normal function of cells and organs. Common electrolytes include sodium, potassium, chloride and bicarbonate. These, together with calcium, magnesium, phosphate and sulphate, can be found in sweat. When we sweat during exercise, we need to replace these electrolytes to keep the electrolyte concentrations of our body fluids constant. Sports drinks contain sodium chloride or potassium chloride as well as sugar and flavourings for extra energy, and to make the drink taste better. Isotonic sports drinks such as Lucozade Sport are preferred by middle-distance to long-distance runners and games players as they replace lost fluids and give a carbohydrate boost. Hypotonic drinks replace lost fluids but do not give a carbohydrate boost. These are used regularly by jockeys and gymnasts who need to keep their weight down. However, there are currently no examples of hypotonic drinks in the UK. You can make your own quite easily using 100 ml of orange or blackcurrant squash, 1 l of water and a pinch of salt; mix and it is ready to serve.

Achieving optimal weight

There are many weight tables available that tell you what your ideal weight should be for your height, but these tables do not take into account your body frame or your age. More accurate weight assessments look at body composition. This means calculating the percentage of body fat and lean body mass. A woman should have no more than 30% body fat and a man no more than 20% body fat.

Optimal weight in sport varies according to activity. Training and dietary choice will affect the amount of muscle mass and body fat. A prop in rugby league will be heavier than a winger because the requirements of these positions are different. Props need a large muscle mass to support the scrum and break through the opposition, whereas wingers tend to be leaner as they need speed to evade the opposition. In boxing, optimal weight is crucial to keep in a certain weight category, while a jockey needs to be light, as excess weight is seen as a handicap.

Training can affect the weight of a performer. Power athletes have a bulky muscle fibre mass through lots of weight training involving heavy weights, whereas endurance performers generally have a very lean look.

Athletes' diets

Appropriate nutrition and diet can contribute to a successful performance. A balanced diet is essential for optimum performance in all sporting activities. What you eat can have an effect on your health, your weight and your energy levels. Top performers place huge demands on their bodies during training and competition. Their diet must meet those energy requirements as well as providing nutrients for tissue growth and repair. An average diet should contain around 15% protein, 30% fat and 55% carbohydrate. During exercise, this percentage needs to change in favour of carbohydrates. Sports nutritionists recommend the following:

Proteins:	10–15%
Fats:	20–25%
Carbohydrates:	60–75%

Diet composition of an endurance athlete versus a power athlete

The body's preferred fuel for any endurance sport is muscle glycogen. If muscle glycogen breakdown exceeds its replacement then glycogen stores become depleted. This results in fatigue and the inability to maintain the duration and intensity of training. In order to replenish and maintain glycogen stores, an endurance athlete needs a diet rich in carbohydrates. Most research seems to suggest that endurance athletes need to consume at least 6–10 grams of carbohydrate per kilogram of body weight. Another key nutrient is water, to avoid dehydration. Some endurance athletes manipulate their diet to maximise aerobic energy production. One method of achieving this is glycogen loading (often called carbo-loading, see pages 30–31).

In general, endurance athletes require more carbohydrates than power athletes simply because they exercise for longer periods of time and need more energy. By contrast, proteins are very important for power athletes. The building blocks of protein are amino acids and although the body can make non-essential amino acids, essential amino acids need to be supplied by diet. Not getting enough protein will lead to muscle breakdown. Proteins are also important for tissue growth and repair and can be a minor source of energy.

Practice makes perfect

1. How does the diet of an endurance athlete differ from that of a power athlete? *(3 marks)*
2. Name one illegal ergogenic aid that would be of benefit to an endurance performer and explain how it can help performance. *(3 marks)*
3. Discuss the advantages and disadvantages of taking creatine and sodium bicarbonate supplements. *(4 marks)*

Chapter 6

Applied physiology to optimise performance

Specialised training

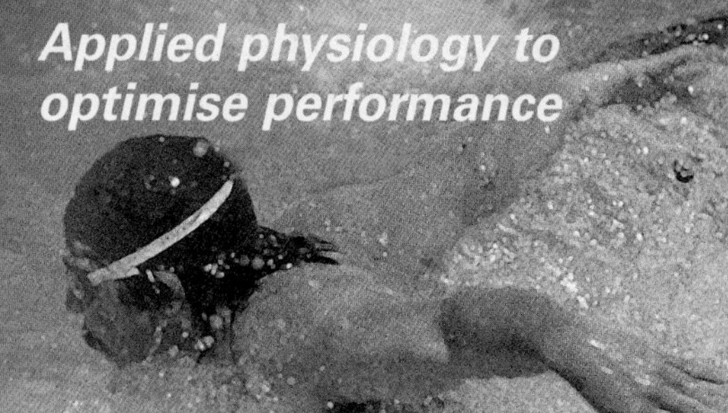

What you need to know

By the end of this chapter, you should be able to:

- understand what each type of specialised training involves
- understand the physiological reasons why a specific type of training is used
- identify which athletes find a particular training method useful and assess whether it is effective

Altitude training

The percentage of oxygen (O_2) in the air is the same at sea level and at altitude. However, the **partial pressure** of oxygen decreases as altitude increases, causing a reduction in the diffusion gradient between the air and the lungs and between the alveoli and the blood. As a result, haemoglobin is not fully saturated at altitude, which results in a lower oxygen-carrying capacity of the blood. As less oxygen is delivered to working muscles there is an earlier onset of fatigue. This results in a decrease in performance (of aerobic activities). However, the body's response to the reduced levels of oxygen provides a number of advantages, as described in Table 6.1.

Table 6.1 Advantages and disadvantages of altitude training

Advantages of altitude training	Disadvantages of altitude training
Increase in the number of red blood cells Increased concentration of haemoglobin Enhanced oxygen transport Effects last for 10–14 days on return to lower altitude so an advantage if a major competition is imminent	Expensive for British athletes due to travel and accommodation costs Altitude sickness Difficult to train due to the lack of oxygen Training intensity has to reduce when the performer first trains at altitude due to the decreased availability of oxygen Benefits can be quickly lost on return to sea level so a disadvantage for regular competitions spread throughout the season

Plyometrics

If leg power is crucial to successful performance, for example in the long jump and 100 m sprint in athletics or rebounding in basketball, then plyometrics is one method of strength

> **Top tip**
> Make sure you can relate plyometrics to the muscle spindle apparatus.

training that will improve the power or elastic strength required. Plyometrics works on the concept that muscles can generate more force if they have previously been stretched. This occurs in plyometrics when, on landing, the muscle performs an eccentric contraction (lengthens under tension). This stimulates the muscle spindle apparatus as it detects the rapid lengthening of the muscle and then sends nerve impulses to the central nervous system (CNS). If the CNS believes the muscle is lengthening too quickly it will initiate a stretch reflex, causing a powerful concentric contraction as the performer jumps up.

To develop leg strength a line of benches, boxes or hurdles is made and the performer has to jump, hop or leap from one to the other. Recovery occurs as the performer walks back to the start line to repeat the exercise.

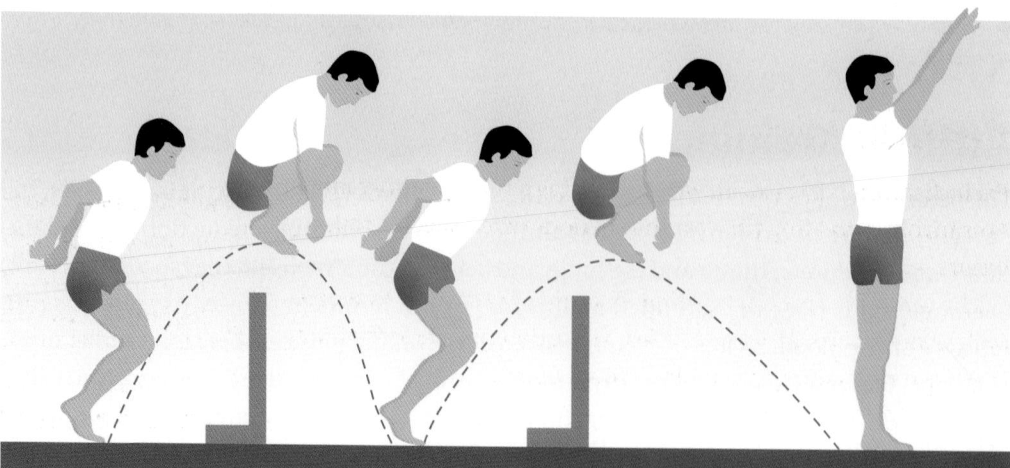

Figure 6.1 Plyometric training

Arm strength can be developed by, for example, performing press-ups with mid-air claps or throwing and catching a medicine ball.

Proprioceptive neuromuscular facilitation (PNF)

Proprioceptive neuromuscular facilitation, or PNF, is an advanced stretching technique. It is considered to be one of the most effective forms of flexibility training for increasing range of motion because it facilitates muscular inhibition. First the muscle should be passively stretched, then contracted isometrically against a resistance while in a stretched position for a period of at least 10 seconds. When it is then passively stretched again there is an increase in the range of motion. PNF stretching tends to be more effective with the help of a partner (see Figure 6.2).

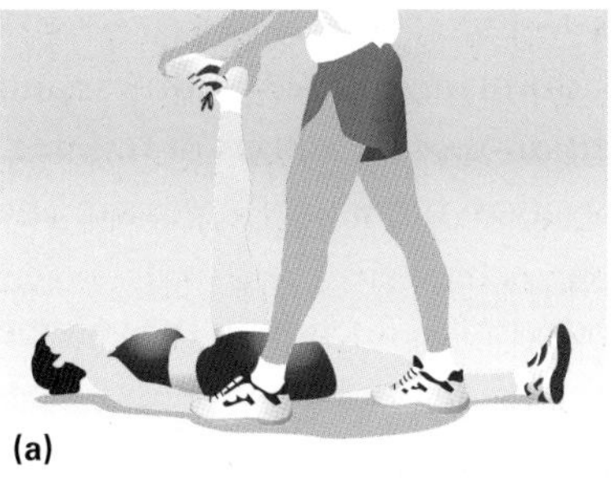
(a)

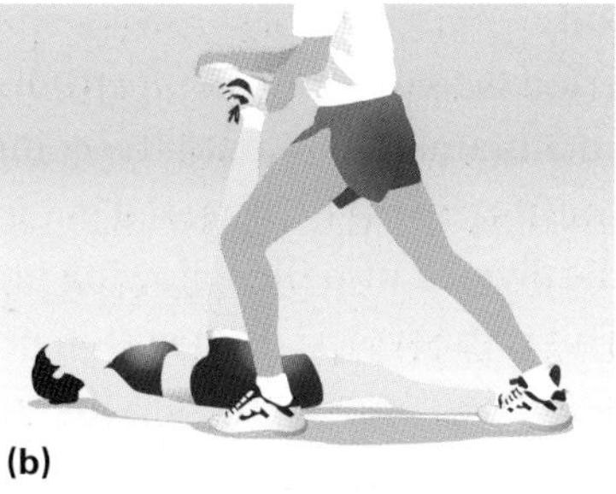
(b)

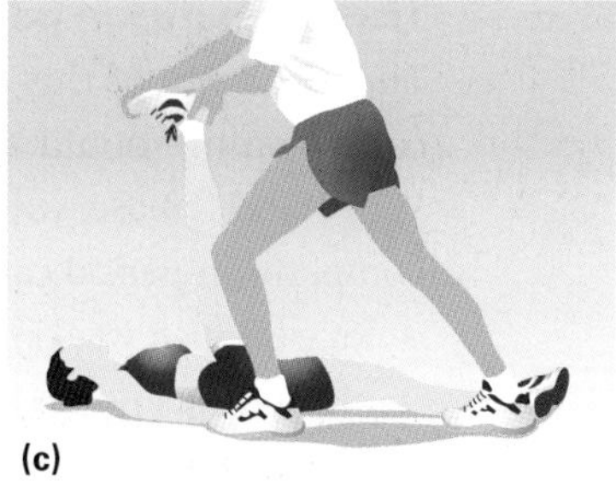
(c)

Figure 6.2 (a) The individual performs a passive stretch with the help of a partner and extends the leg until tension is felt. This stretch is detected by the muscle spindle apparatus.
(b) The individual then isometrically contracts the muscle for at least 10 seconds by pushing his/her leg against the partner, who supplies just enough resistance to hold the leg in a stationary position. Golgi tendon organs are sensitive to tension developed in a muscle. During an isometric contraction they send an inhibitory signal which overrides the excitatory signal from the muscle spindle and delays the stretch reflex.
(c) There is further relaxation of the target muscle as a result and it can be stretched further during the next passive stretch.

Periodisation

Periodisation is a key word when planning a training programme. This involves dividing the year into periods when specific training occurs.

The seasonal approach is now commonly adapted to macrocycles, mesocycles and microcycles. These describe periods of time that are more prescriptive for individual needs.

> **Key term**
> **Periodisation:** dividing the training year into specific sections for a specific purpose.

> **Tasks to tackle 6.1**
> Using your own sport, list the activities that you would do during the following periods:
> Off season
> Pre-season
> Competitive season

Macrocycle

The macrocycle — the 'big' period — involves a long-term performance goal. For a footballer this may be the length of the season while for athletes it could be 4 years as they build up to the Olympic Games. The macrocycle is made up of three distinct periods.

The preparation period

This is often referred to as pre-season training and is divided into:

- Phase 1 — general conditioning training. This should consist of a lot of low-intensity work. Athletes should aim to develop aerobic and muscular endurance, general strength and mobility.
- Phase 2 — competition-specific training. This involves an increase in the intensity of training. During this time, strength and speed work should be done. This phase also introduces technique and tactical work, so that the performer is prepared for the start of the competitive season.

The competition period

The main aim of this period is to optimise competition performance. Levels of fitness and conditioning should be maintained, as should the competition-specific aspects of training. Within this phase, volume of training is decreased but intensity of training is increased. The competition period can be divided into the following phases:

- Phase 3 (6–8 weeks). This is the typical competition period with a reduction in the volume of training and an increase in competition-specific training. Trials and qualifying competitions fall within this phase.
- Phase 4 (4–6 weeks). During a long competitive season it is a good idea to have a mini period where competitions are kept to a minimum or eliminated altogether and the level of competition-specific training is reduced. This allows the body to recover and prepare for phase 5.
- Phase 5 (3–4 weeks). This is the end of the training year when all the major events and competitions fall, for example a football cup final or the Commonwealth Games. Competition-specific training is maintained and tapering should occur.

Tapering is a reduction in the volume of training prior to major competition. This allows the athlete to reach peak performance. It is important for the coach to ensure that peak performance occurs in a certain time span so the performer can benefit from the removal of training-induced fatigue but reversibility has not yet come into effect. A typical taper will last between 10 and 21 days but can vary between different sports and performers.

The transition or recovery period

This is phase 6, the final phase of the year, and involves recovery. This phase allows the athlete to recharge physically and mentally and ensures an injury-free start to the following season. General, fun exercise should be carried out during this phase.

Mesocycle

This describes a short-term goal within the macrocycle, which may last for 2–8 weeks. This cycle may have a component of fitness as the focus, for example a sprinter will focus on power, reaction time and speed, whereas an endurance performer will focus more on strength endurance and cardio-respiratory endurance.

Microcycle

This is normally just a description of 1 week of training that is repeated throughout the length of the mesocycle. It could set out what the performer is going to do on each day from Monday to Sunday, including rest days (usually in a 3:1 ratio).

The training unit

This is a description of one training session, which will be following a key training objective.

Tasks to tackle 6.2

Using a copy of the table below, describe what activities you might do to satisfy the aims of the session.

Training aim	Details of training session
A session to improve lactate tolerance	
A session to improve strength in the upper body	

Double periodisation

Some sports require an athlete to peak more than once in a season. A long-distance athlete, for example, may want to peak in winter during the cross-country season and then again in the summer on the track. An international footballer may want to peak for an important cup final for his club and for a cup competition later in the year for his country. In this case, these performers have to follow a double-periodised year.

Lactate sampling

Blood lactate measurements are used by elite performers in sports such as running, swimming and rowing to monitor training and predict performance. The measurements are used as a means of measuring training intensity, while the higher the pace at which the lactate threshold occurs, the fitter the athlete is considered to be. Lactate sampling allows the performer to select relevant training zones — expressed in terms of heart rate (beats per minute) or power (watts) — in order to get the desired training effect.

Regular lactate testing provides a comparison from which the coach and performer can see whether improvement has occurred. If test results increase, this indicates that the performer has an increase in peak speed/power, increased time to exhaustion, improved recovery heart rate and, finally, a higher lactate threshold.

Respiratory exchange ratio (RER)

Energy sources such as carbohydrates, fats and proteins can all be oxidised to produce energy. For a certain volume of oxygen, the energy released will depend on the energy source.

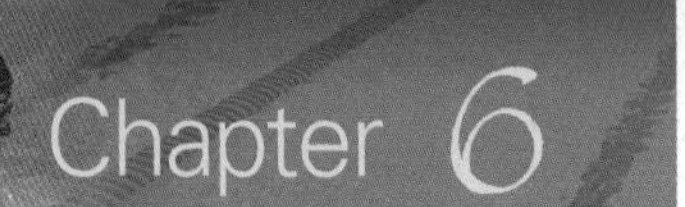

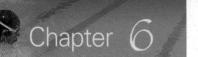

Calculating the respiratory exchange ratio (RER) will determine which of these energy sources is being oxidised. RER is the ratio of carbon dioxide produced to oxygen consumed. It is also referred to as the respiratory quotient (RQ).

- An RER value of 0.7 indicates that the predominant fuel source is fat.
- An RER value of 0.8–0.9 indicates that the source is a mix of fats and carbohydrates.
- An RER value of 1.0 indicates that the predominant fuel source is carbohydrate.

Practice makes perfect

1 Many coaches plan the year using a technique called periodisation. Explain what is meant by periodisation. *(4 marks)*

2 What do you understand by the term respiratory exchange ratio? *(3 marks)*

3 Explain the role of the muscle spindle apparatus in plyometrics. *(3 marks)*

Chapter 7

Applied physiology to optimise performance

Sports injuries

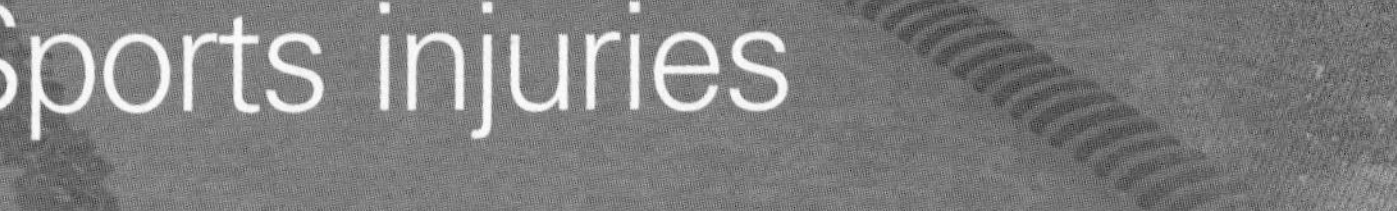

What you need to know

By the end of this chapter you should be able to:

- state what hyperbaric chambers, oxygen tents and ice baths are
- understand the physiological reasons for their use
- state which athletes find them useful
- decide whether each is effective
- define DOMS and explain why it occurs

> Key term
>
> **RICE:** rest, ice, compression, elevation.

Most common sporting injuries tend to be muscle strains, often caused by performers going too hard or too fast in their activity. Treatment for these injuries is simply **RICE** (rest, ice, compression, elevation).

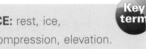

Overuse injuries, resulting from excessive wear and tear on the muscles and joints, also occur frequently. Typical overuse injuries include 'runners knee', shin splints and 'tennis elbow'. These injuries, depending on their severity, can be treated with RICE, cortisone injections or, in some cases, surgery.

More serious injuries, such as fractures, require longer treatment and can put professional athletes out of action for long periods of time. A fracture is a break in a bone. Overuse can also cause stress fractures, which are very small cracks in a bone.

A common football fracture is that of the metatarsals, the bones in the feet. Players such as David Beckham, Wayne Rooney, Steven Gerrard, Michael Owen and Gary Neville have all experienced this injury and received high-tech treatment, including the use of hyperbaric chambers.

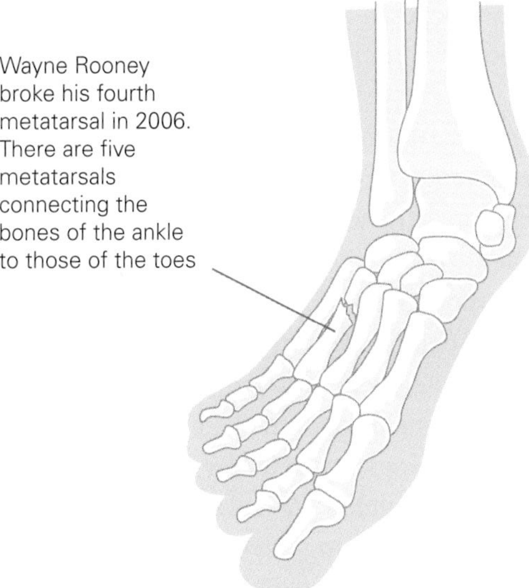

Wayne Rooney broke his fourth metatarsal in 2006. There are five metatarsals connecting the bones of the ankle to those of the toes

Figure 7.1 Location of the metatarsals

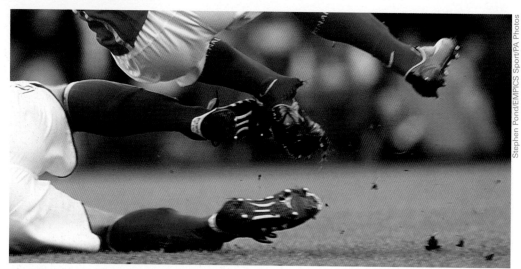
Stephen Pond/EMPICS Sport/PA Photos

Arsenal's Eduardo Da Silva received a broken leg when he was tackled by Birmingham City's Martin Taylor. Taylor was sent off for the offence.

Prevention and rehabilitation

Hyperbaric chambers

The aim of hyperbaric chambers is to reduce the recovery time for an injury. The chamber is pressurised rather like an aeroplane (in some chambers, a mask is worn). The pressure increases the amount of oxygen that can be breathed in and this means more oxygen can be diffused to the injured area. The dissolved oxygen can reduce swelling and stimulate the body's cells to repair. Many sportsmen and women use hyperbaric chambers. Wayne Rooney, for example, used a hyperbaric chamber before the 2006 football World Cup to try to speed up recovery from his broken metatarsal.

Oxygen tents

Oxygen tents are also known as hypoxic tents. Elite sportsmen and women may sleep in them overnight as the tents simulate the effects of high altitude by providing a low-oxygen environment. The oxygen depletion causes production of higher levels of haemoglobin, which means more oxygen can be extracted from the blood for extra energy. Oxygen tents do not make a difference to the speed of the healing process but do mean that when the performers have recovered from injury, they will have retained a level of fitness that allows them to return to their sport almost immediately.

The tents are very useful for endurance activities such as cycling, or sports that require a high level of stamina, such as football. Lance Armstrong, the celebrated Tour de France cyclist, used one as a training device and the technique is now common among the cycling elite, although controversial. David Beckham famously used one before the 2002 football World Cup to maintain high levels of fitness while he recovered from injury.

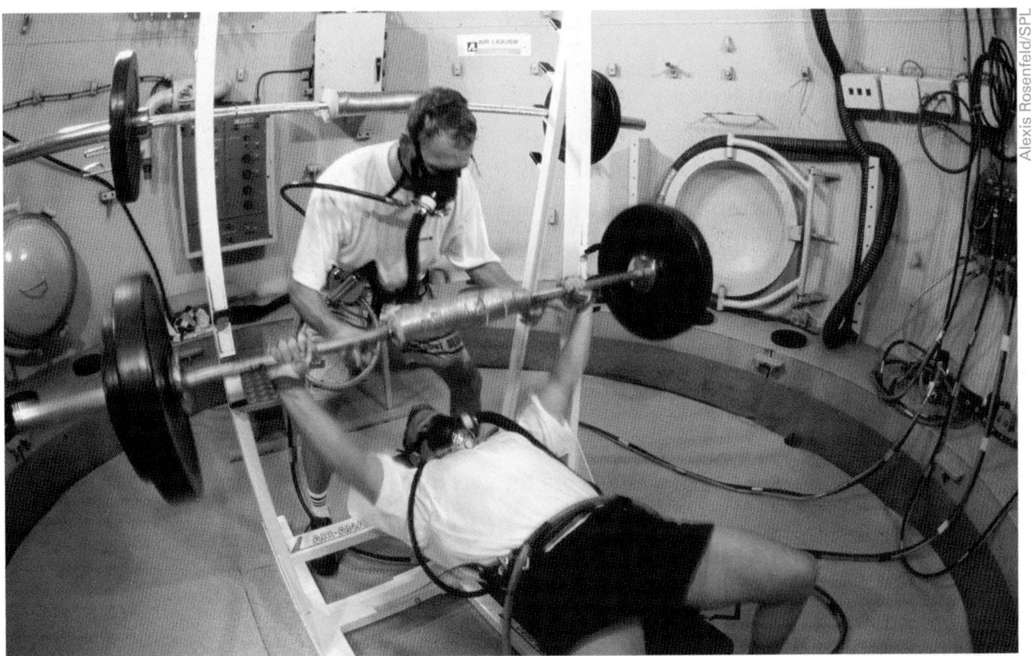
Alexis Rosenfeld/SPL

A hyperbaric chamber

Ice baths

Ice baths are a very popular recovery method. After a gruelling training session or match, sports performers get into an ice bath for 5–10 minutes. The cold water causes the blood vessels to tighten and drains the blood out of the legs. The blood that leaves the legs takes away with it the lactic acid that has built up during the activity. On leaving the bath, the legs fill up with new blood that invigorates the muscles with oxygen to help the cells function better.

Ice baths are now used by most professional sportsmen and women who train and play regularly. Most rugby Super League teams do 'hot and cold' sessions, where players spend 2 minutes in the steam room followed by 1 minute in the cold plunge pool. The purpose is to flush lactic acid from the muscles, reducing soreness for the week ahead. Despite its unpleasantness, the benefits can be felt immediately, especially in the legs. Some players include 'hot and colds' in their pre-match routine on game day.

DOMS

One aim of training is to improve fitness levels. An individual who wishes to improve strength will often work at higher intensities to overload the muscle in order to stimulate muscle hypertrophy. When this occurs the individual may experience tender and painful muscles some 24–48 hours after exercise. This is called DOMS or **delayed onset of muscle soreness**.

Top tip

Make sure you know which athletes find these recovery methods useful.

This muscle soreness is a result of structural damage to muscle fibres and connective tissue surrounding the fibres. DOMS usually occurs following excessive eccentric contraction when muscle fibres are put under a lot of strain. This type of muscular contraction is performed mostly during weight training and plyometrics.

A thorough warm-up and cool-down can help to avoid the delayed soreness or, at the very least, keep it to a minimum. If eccentric muscle contractions are the major causal factor, training should try to minimise the use of these or at least ensure training intensity is increased gradually.

Practice makes perfect

1 What do you understand by the term DOMS? *(3 marks)*

2 How do hyperbaric chambers help in the rehabilitation of sports injuries? *(3 marks)*

3 Ice baths are increasingly used by sports performers as a recovery aid. How does an ice bath help a performer to recover? *(3 marks)*

Chapter 8

Applied physiology to optimise performance

Mechanics of movement

What you need to know

By the end of this chapter you should be able to:

- understand vectors and scalars in relation to acceleration, momentum and impulse in sprinting
- describe Newton's laws and apply them to movements
- understand the application of forces in sporting activities
- understand projectile motion, including the factors affecting distance and vector components of parabolic flight
- understand the concept of angular motion and how it is conserved during flight
- describe the moment of inertia and explain its relationship with angular velocity

This chapter looks at developing your knowledge of the mechanics of movement and shows how applying this to sporting activities can facilitate the development and enhancement of performance.

Linear motion

Linear motion is motion in a straight or curved line, with all body parts moving the same distance at the same speed in the same direction. In tobogganing, for example, the toboggan moves in a straight line. In the shot put, the shot moves in a curved line.

There are several mechanical concepts involved with linear motion.

Newton's laws of motion

Newton's first law of motion (the law of inertia):

A body continues in its state of rest or motion in a straight line, unless compelled to change that state by external forces exerted upon it.

Newton's second law of motion (the law of acceleration):

The rate of change of momentum of a body (or the acceleration for a body of constant mass) is proportional to the force causing it and the change that takes place in the direction in which the force acts.

Newton's third law of motion (the law of reaction):

To every action there is an equal and opposite reaction.

Table 8.1 applies these laws to football.

Table 8.1 The application of Newton's laws to football

Newton's laws	Application
Law of inertia	In a penalty kick, the ball (body) will remain on the spot (in a state of rest) until it is kicked by the player (an external force is exerted upon it).
Law of acceleration	When the player kicks (force applied) the ball during the game, the acceleration of the ball (rate of change of momentum) is proportional to the size of the force. So, the harder the ball is kicked the further and faster it will go.
Law of reaction	When a footballer jumps up (action) to win a header, a force is exerted on the ground in order to gain height. At the same time the ground exerts an upward force (equal and opposite reaction) upon the footballer.

Tasks to tackle 8.1

Copy and complete the table below giving an example of how each of the laws can be applied to a sport of your choice.

Newton's laws	Application
Law of inertia	
Law of acceleration	
Law of reaction	

The measurements used in linear motion

The measurements used in linear motion are listed below. Knowledge of these will help in your understanding of mechanics and motion:

- mass
- inertia
- distance
- speed
- weight
- acceleration
- deceleration
- displacement
- velocity
- momentum

These measurements can be split into two groups:

- **Scalar quantities** are described in terms of size or magnitude — mass, inertia, distance and speed are scalar quantities.

- **Vector quantities** are described in terms of size and direction — weight, acceleration, deceleration, displacement, velocity and momentum are vector quantities.

Mass versus weight

Mass is a physical quantity expressing the amount of matter in a body. Our mass is made up of bone, muscle, fat, tissue and fluid and is measured in kilograms. A sumo wrestler, for example, has a much greater mass than a gymnast. Mass is a scalar quantity because it does not have direction, just size.

Weight is the force on a given mass due to gravity. As the strength of gravity is the same everywhere on the surface of the Earth, the gravitational force exerted on an object (its weight) is directly proportional to its mass. So, if the sumo wrestler has a mass, for example, three times as much as the gymnast, then the sumo wrestler's weight is three times that of the gymnast. This means that an object's mass can be measured indirectly by its weight. However, the strength of gravity is different on the moon, for example, where it is one-sixth of that on the Earth. So if a gymnast has a mass of 40 kg, this stays the same on the moon, but his/her weight would be one-sixth less. Weight is a vector quantity because it has both size and direction — weight acts downwards from the centre of mass. Weight is a unit of force and is measured in newtons.

Inertia

Inertia is the resistance an object has to a change in its state of motion. If an object is at rest it will remain still. If it is moving in one direction it will continue to do so at the same speed until another force is exerted upon it (see Newton's first law). The bigger the mass, the larger the inertia of the body or object. This means that more force will be needed to change its state of motion. Consider two rugby league players running towards you. One is a prop weighing 100 kg and the other a winger weighing 75 kg; which one would you prefer to stop? The winger will be easier to stop because he has less inertia. Only the very brave would attempt to stop the prop!

Distance versus displacement

Distance and displacement are quantities that are used to describe the extent of a body's motion. **Distance** is the length of the path a body follows when moving from one position to another. For example, a 200 m runner who has just completed a race has run a distance of 200 m as shown in Figure 8.1. This is a scalar quantity because it just measures size.

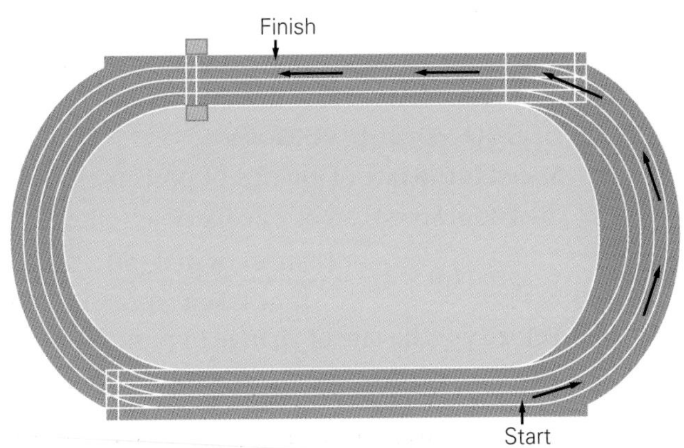

Figure 8.1 The distance of a 200 m race

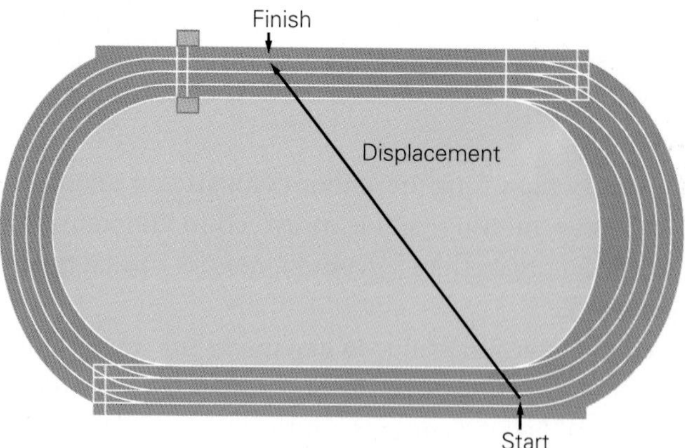

Figure 8.2 The displacement of a 200 m race

Displacement is the length of a straight line joining the start and finish points. For example, in a 200 m race on a track the length of the path the athlete follows (distance) is 200 m but his/her displacement will be the number of metres as the crow flies from the start to the finish (Figure 8.2).

Displacement is a vector quantity because it describes both size and direction. Figure 8.3 shows a javelin throw and a basketball free throw to further illustrate the difference between distance and displacement.

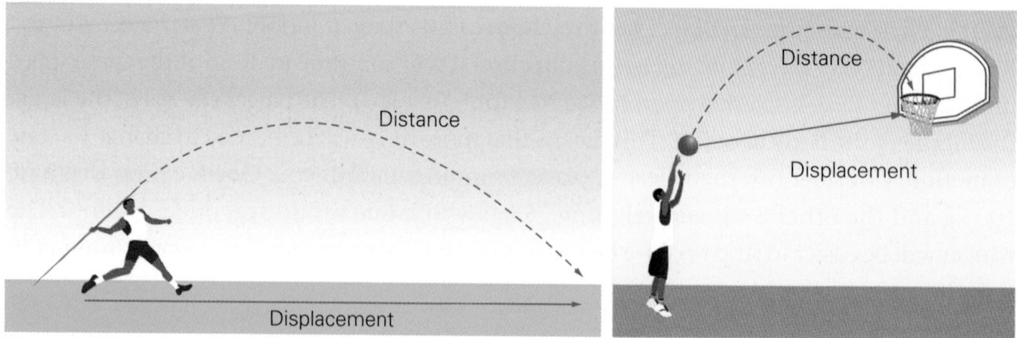

Figure 8.3 More examples of distance and displacement

Speed versus velocity

Speed is the rate of change of position. It is a scalar quantity because it does not consider direction. Speed can be calculated as follows:

$$\text{speed (m s}^{-1}\text{)} = \frac{\text{distance covered (m)}}{\text{time taken (s)}}$$

Velocity is the rate of change of position with reference to direction. This means that it is a more precise description of motion and is a vector quantity. It can be calculated as follows:

$$\text{velocity (m s}^{-1}\text{)} = \frac{\text{displacement (m)}}{\text{time taken (s)}}$$

Tasks to tackle 8.2

(a) Work out the displacement of the following components of a triathlon:

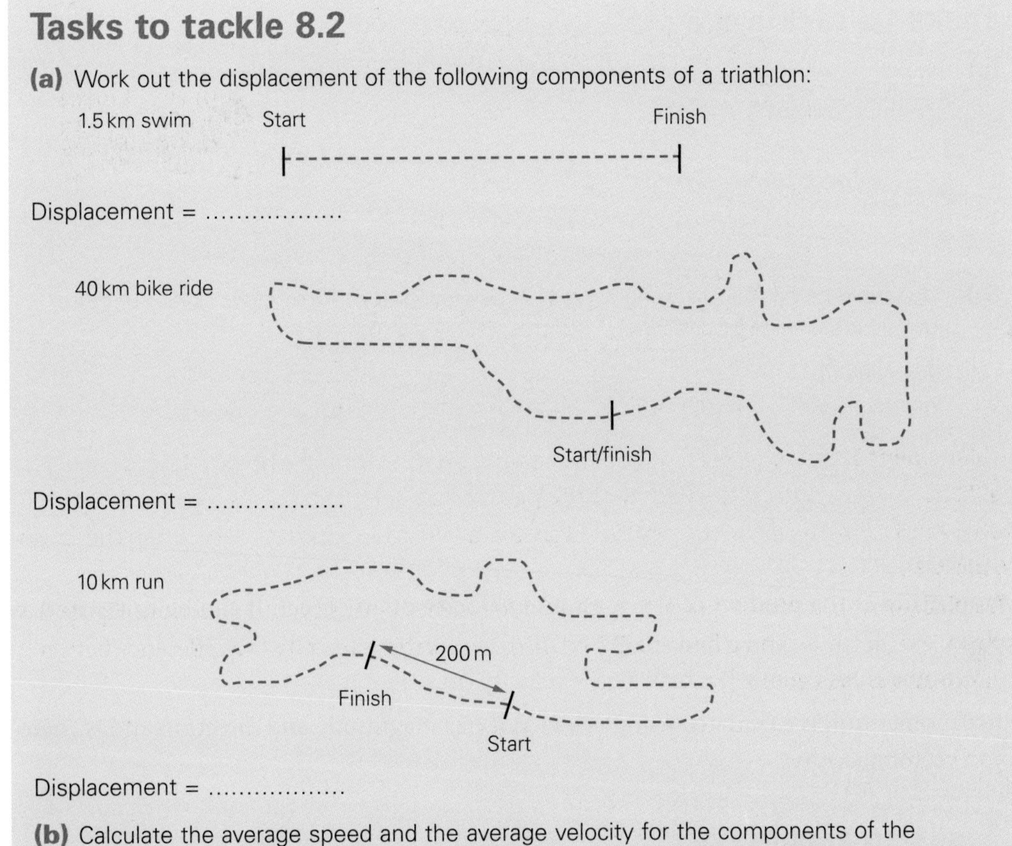

(b) Calculate the average speed and the average velocity for the components of the triathlon.

Distance	Time	Displacement	Average speed	Average velocity
1.5 km swim	30 min 30 s			
40 km cycle	90 min			
10 km run	45 min			

Acceleration and deceleration

These can both be defined as the rate of change of velocity. **Acceleration** occurs when velocity increases and **deceleration** occurs when velocity decreases. They are vector quantities.

Acceleration can be calculated as follows:

$$\text{acceleration} = \frac{\text{change in velocity (m s}^{-1}\text{)}}{\text{time taken (s)}}$$

To calculate the change in velocity the following equation is used:

$$\text{change in velocity} = \frac{V_f - V_i}{t} = \frac{\text{final velocity} - \text{initial velocity}}{\text{time}}$$

Tasks to tackle 8.3

(a) Think of three examples in any team game where acceleration and/or deceleration are important quantities.

1 ....

2 ....

3 ....

(b) In the table below, calculate the average acceleration of a 100 m runner over 20-metre intervals (no change of direction).

Distance (m)	0	20	40	60	80	100
Velocity (m s^{-1})	0.00	8.5	11.1	11.5	11.5	9.5
Time (s)	0.0	2.9	5.6	7.6	9.4	11.4
Acceleration	N/A					

Momentum

Momentum is the product of the mass and velocity of an object. It can be calculated as follows:

momentum (kg m s^{-1}) = mass (kg) × velocity (m s^{-1})

Since momentum is calculated using velocity, it has magnitude and direction and is therefore a vector quantity.

Tasks to tackle 8.4

Complete the blanks in the table below.

Performer	Mass (kg)	Velocity (m s^{-1})	Momentum (kg m s^{-1})
100 m sprinter	80	10.0	
Prop	105		893
Centre forward	70	9.5	
Middle-distance runner	65		585

From the table in task 8.4 it can be seen that a large mass, coupled with the ability to run at a high velocity, results in a high momentum. If you had to stop any of the performers listed, the prop would be the most difficult as his momentum is the greatest.

In a closed system, total momentum is conserved. So when two objects collide, for example, the total momentum stays the same, although some may transfer from one object to the other. Most sporting situations, however, are not closed systems. For example, when a cricket bat hits the ball, the ball is squashed to a degree. After a few milliseconds, it rebounds back. This contraction and rebound action causes the release of heat energy, and some momentum is lost.

Force

A **force** can be described as a 'push' or 'pull'. It can cause a body at rest to move or cause a moving body to stop, slow down, speed up or change direction. Forces can be either internal or external. Internal forces are generated through the contraction of skeletal muscle, whereas external forces come from outside the body, for example air resistance, friction, weight and reaction. It is important to consider the following when describing a force:

- The size or magnitude of the force — this is dependent on the size and number of muscle fibres used.
- The direction of the force — if a force is applied through the middle of an object it will move in the same direction as the force, as shown in Figure 8.4.

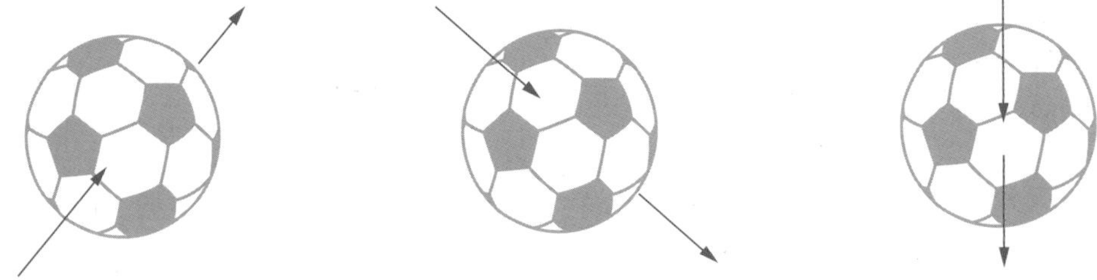

Figure 8.4 A central force gives movement in the same direction as the force

- The position of application of force — this is an important factor in sport. Applying a force straight through the centre results in movement in a straight line (linear motion), as shown in Figure 8.5. Applying a force off-centre results in spin (angular momentum), as shown in Figure 8.6.

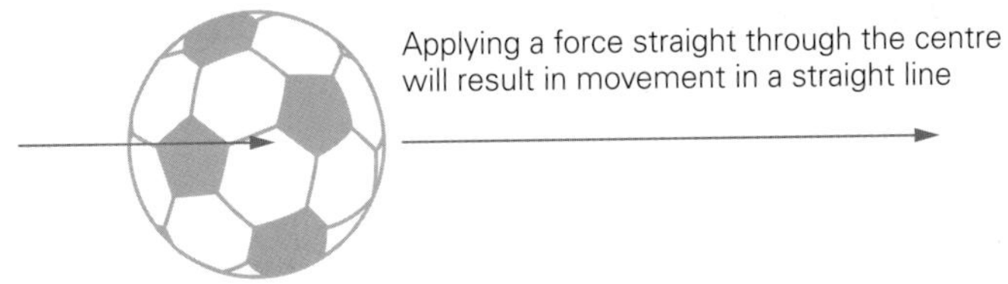
Applying a force straight through the centre
will result in movement in a straight line

Figure 8.5 A central force gives straight-line movement

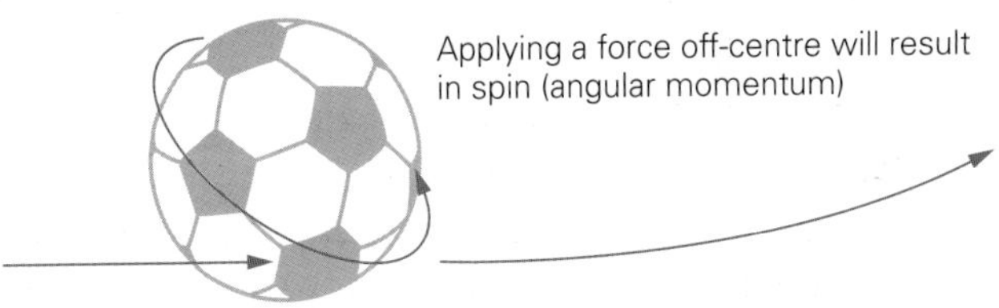
Applying a force off-centre will result
in spin (angular momentum)

Figure 8.6 An off-centre force gives spin

As force is a vector quantity, an arrow can be used to represent it.

Tasks to tackle 8.5

(a) Look at the following pictures and decide where the force is being applied (point of application). Mark this position with a cross.

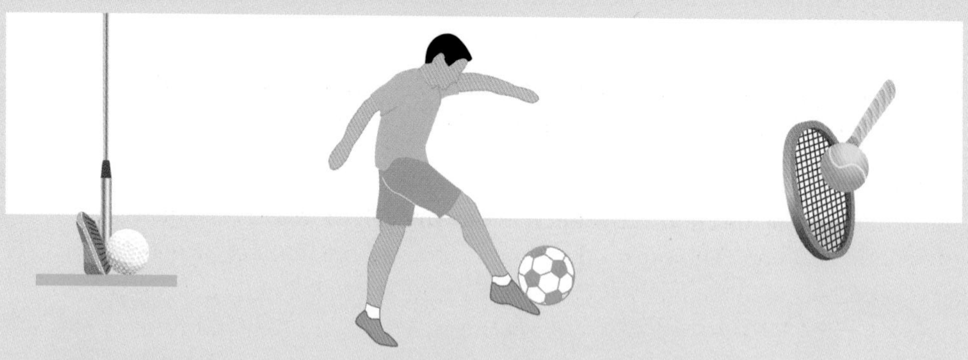

(b) Now label the direction in which the force is acting. Use an arrow starting at the point of application and then draw it in the direction you think the force is acting.

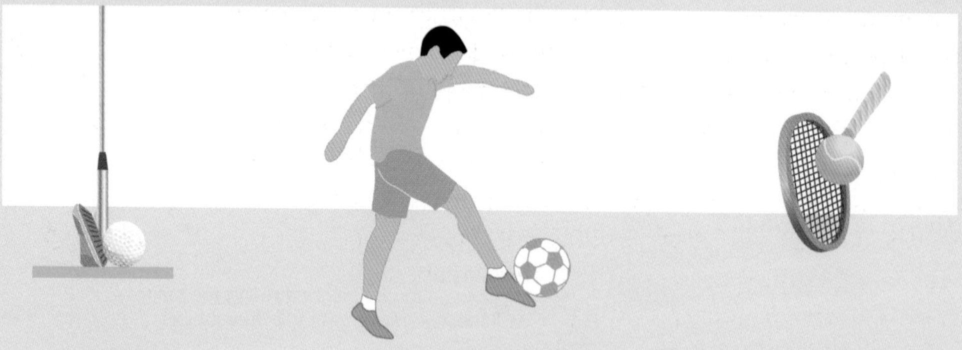

(c) Finally decide how big this force is. The larger the force, the bigger the arrow.

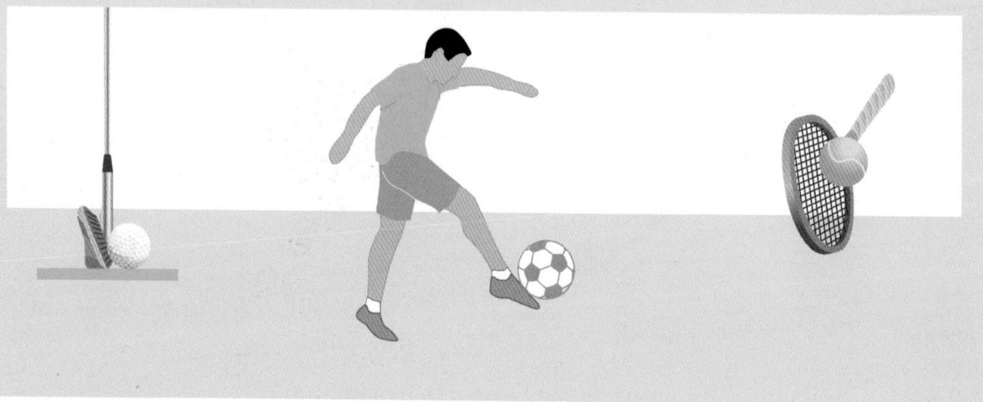

Types of force acting upon a sports performer

Both vertical and horizontal forces act upon a sports performer. Vertical forces are weight and reaction and horizontal forces are friction and air resistance.

Vertical forces

Weight

Remember, weight is a gravitational force that the Earth exerts on a body, pulling it towards the centre of the Earth (or, effectively, downwards).

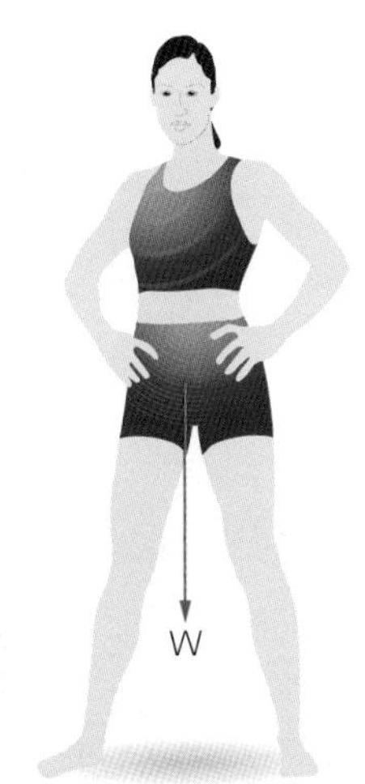

Figure 8.7 Weight

Reaction force

Remember Newton's third law of motion: 'For every action there is an equal and opposite reaction'. This means that there is always a reaction force whenever two bodies are in contact with one another. In Figure 8.8 there are two reaction forces (R), one from the stick on the ball and the other from the ground to the foot. The ground reaction force is a vertical force.

Horizontal forces

Friction

Friction occurs whenever there are two bodies in contact with each other that may have a tendency to slip or slide over each other. Friction acts in opposition to motion. Try to remember that friction resists the slipping or sliding motion of two surfaces. Therefore, in diagrams, a friction arrow is drawn in the opposite direction from this slipping. Usually, this means that a friction arrow points in the same direction as motion, as in Figure 8.9(a). However, in skiing, where the slipping occurs in a forward direction, the friction arrow is reversed as in Figure 8.9(b).

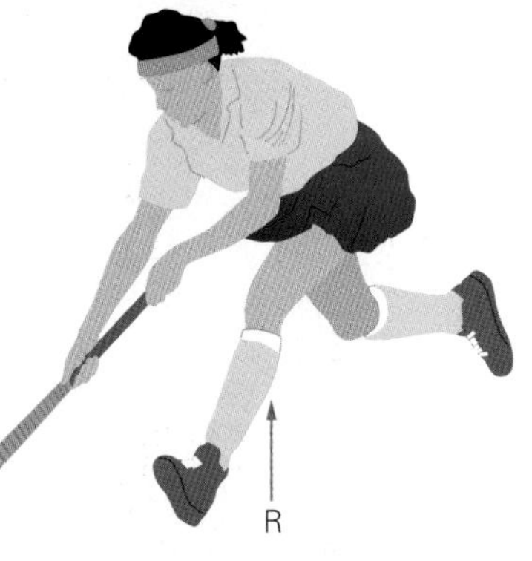

Figure 8.8 Reaction force

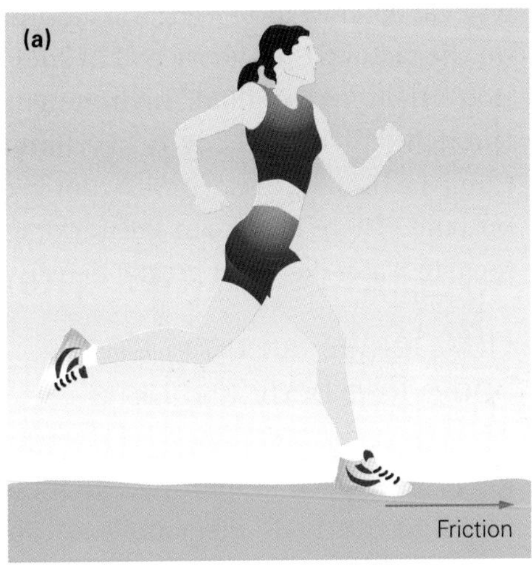

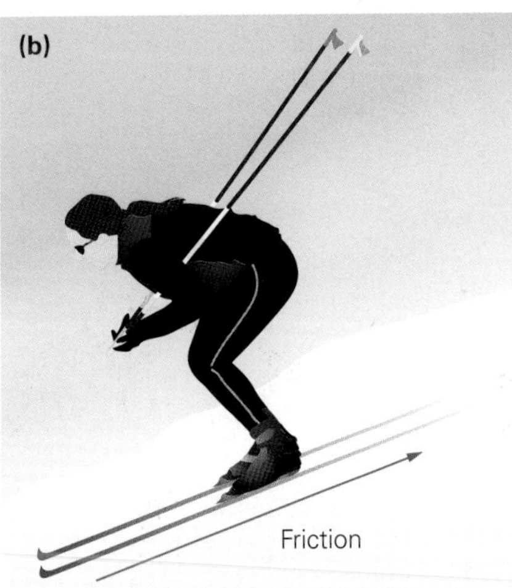

Figure 8.9 Friction opposes the slippage between objects. For a runner (a), the possible slippage of the feet is backwards so the friction arrow points forwards. For a skier (b), the slippage is forwards, so the friction arrow points backwards

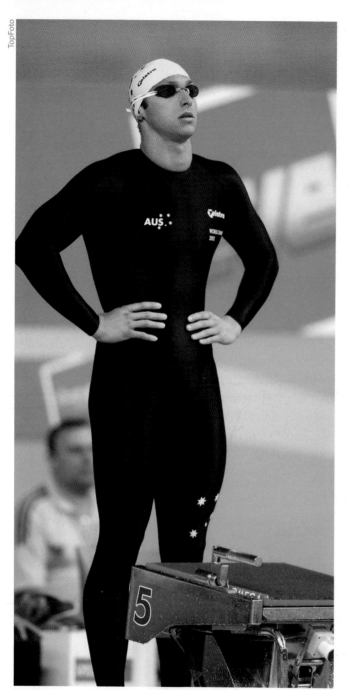

TopFoto

Most elite swimmers shave off all body hair to create a smooth surface; many wear a swimming cap for the same reason. More recently, swimmers have started to wear 'shark suits', or full-body swimsuits, to streamline their surface.

Air resistance and drag

Air resistance opposes the motion of a body travelling through the air. Imagine trying to run into a strong head wind — this is not an easy task as the force of the wind is trying to push you backwards in the opposite direction. Air resistance depends upon:

- the velocity of the moving body — a greater velocity results in a greater resistance
- the cross-sectional area of the moving body — the larger the cross-sectional area, the greater the air resistance. For example, think of how Tour de France competitors reduce their cross-sectional area by crouching low over the handlebars, rather than sitting upright.
- the shape and the surface characteristics of the moving body — a streamlined shape results in less resistance, as does a smooth surface

Air resistance is sometimes referred to as **drag**. Drag is more commonly used to describe the force opposing motion in water as opposed to air. Drag will depend on the factors listed above and in addition the type of fluid environment through which the body is travelling. Compare running in water with running on land. There is a much greater drag force in water due to its greater density.

How forces act upon the body: free body diagrams

For your exam, you need to know how forces are applied in sporting activities. By using free body diagrams you can

The weight force is always drawn down from the centre of mass.	The reaction force starts from where two bodies are in contact with one another. This contact can be the foot with the ground, which is therefore drawn in an upward direction, or can be the contact between sports equipment and a ball such as a tennis racket and a tennis ball.	The friction force starts from where the two bodies are in contact and is opposite to the direction of any potential slipping. It is usually drawn in the same direction as motion.	Air resistance is drawn from the centre of mass opposing the direction of motion of the body.
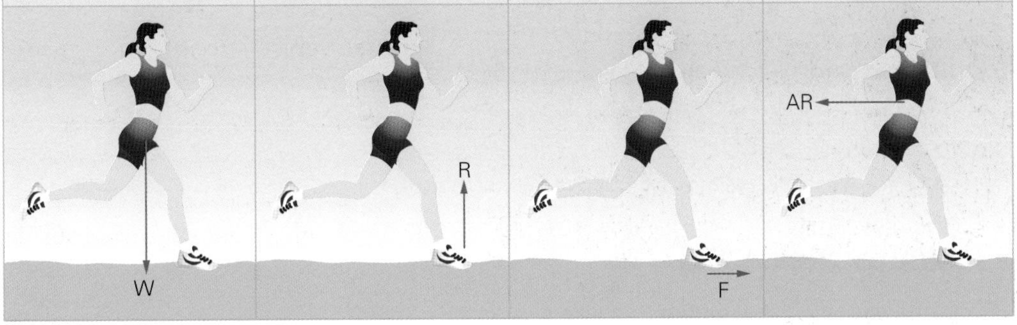 W	R	F	AR

Figure 8.10 Free body diagrams

show the forces acting on a body in the form of an arrow. The longer the arrow, the bigger the size of the force (Figure 8.10).

Net force

This is the resultant force acting on a body when all other forces have been considered. Net force is often discussed in terms of balance versus unbalanced forces.

A **balanced force** is when there are two or more forces acting on a body that are equal in size but opposite in direction. In this case there is zero net force, and therefore no change in the state of motion. This is illustrated in Figure 8.11.

An **unbalanced force** is when a force acting in one direction on a body is larger than the force acting in the opposite direction. This is illustrated in Figure 8.12.

Similarly, if the friction force is equal in length to air resistance then the net result is

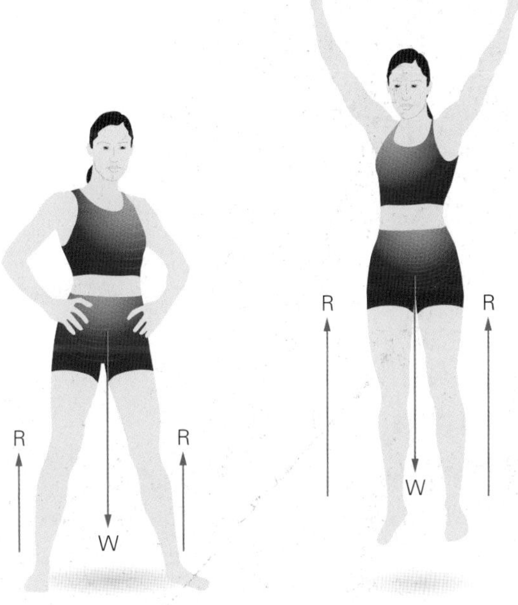

Figure 8.11 When standing, the weight force and reaction force are equal in size but opposite in direction

Figure 8.12 When jumping in the air, the performer accelerates upwards because the reaction force is bigger than the weight force

zero. If the friction arrow is longer than the air resistance arrow, the body will accelerate. If the friction arrow is shorter than the air resistance arrow, the body will decelerate.

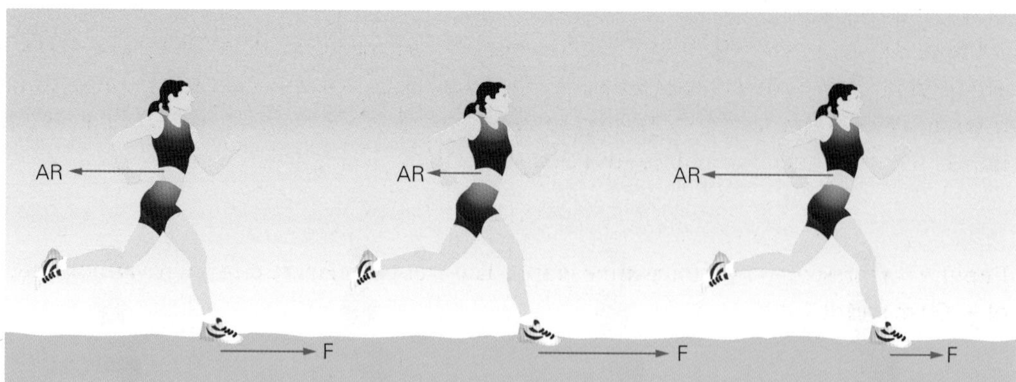

Figure 8.13 $F = AR$ so the net force is 0 $F > AR$ = acceleration $F < AR$ = deceleration

Tasks to tackle 8.6

Label the relevant forces on the following diagrams.

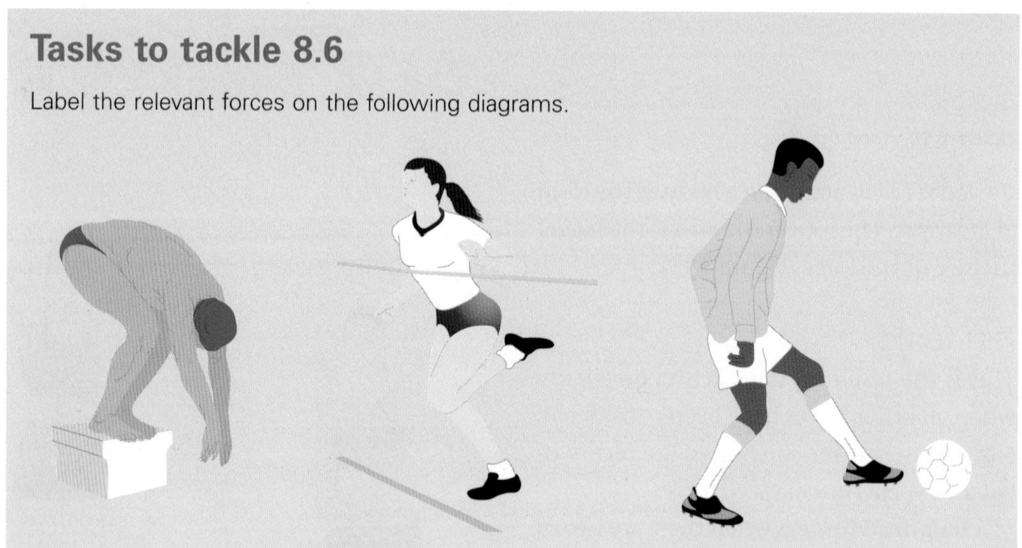

Impulse

Impulse is the product of the average magnitude of a force acting on a body and the time for which that force acts. It is equivalent to the change in the momentum of a body as a result of a force acting on it. Impulse can be calculated as follows:

impulse (newton seconds/N s) = force × time

In a sporting environment, impulse can be used to add speed to a body or object, or to slow it down on impact. Speeding up a body or object can be achieved by increasing the amount of muscular force that is applied. In basketball, for example, a large force is generated when jumping for a rebound in order to get as much height as quickly as possible to catch the ball.

Speeding up a body or object can also be achieved by increasing the amount of time for which the force is applied. In the hammer throw, for example, three to four turns are used as opposed to just a single swing.

Impulse is used to slow down an object or body by increasing the time during which forces act upon it. In any activity that involves a landing action, such as a gymnast dismounting from the parallel bars, flexion of the hip, knee and ankle occurs which extends the time of the impact force and therefore reduces the chance of injury.

Graphical representation of impulse

Impulse is represented by a force–time graph. The graphs in Figure 8.14 show various stages of a 100 m sprint.

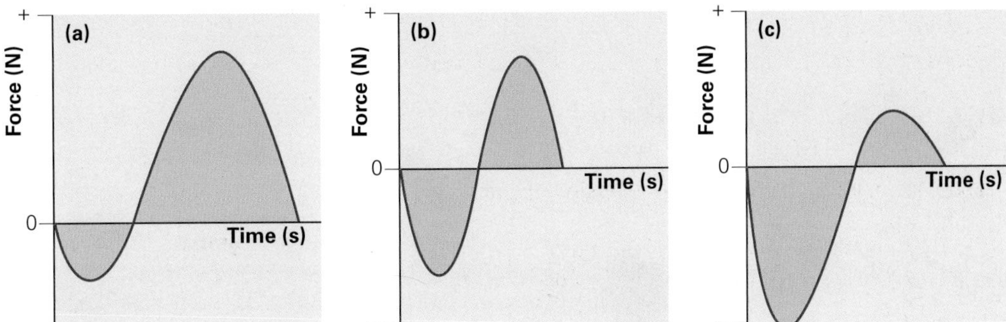

Figure 8.14 (a) Start of the race — the net impulse is positive, which shows that the sprinter is accelerating (b) Middle of the race — the positive and negative impulses are equal (net impulse zero), which means that there is no acceleration or deceleration, so the sprinter is running at a constant velocity (c) End of the race — the net impulse is negative, which shows that the sprinter is decelerating

It is important to note that in running and sprinting, positive impulse occurs for acceleration at take-off, whereas negative impulse occurs when the foot lands to provide a braking action.

Key term

Net impulse: a combination of positive and negative impulses.

Projectile motion

This refers to the motion of either an object or the human body being 'projected' into the air at an angle. We do this all the time in sport, either with a ball or with the human body as a projectile, for example in the long jump and gymnastic vault.

Factors affecting distance

Three factors determine the horizontal distance that a projectile can travel.

Angle of release

To achieve maximum horizontal distance, the angle of release of the projectile is important. This optimum angle of release is dependent upon release height and landing height. When

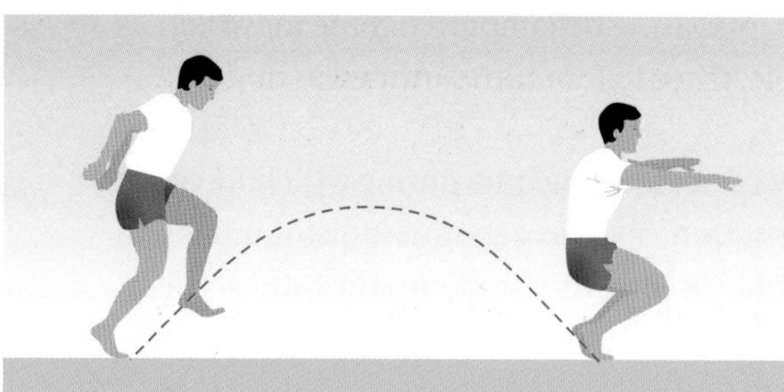
Figure 8.15

both the release height and the landing height are equal then the optimum angle of release is 45°. This would be the case for a long jumper, as in Figure 8.15.

If the release height is greater than the landing height, the optimum angle of release is less than 45°. This can be seen in the shot put, as in Figure 8.16.

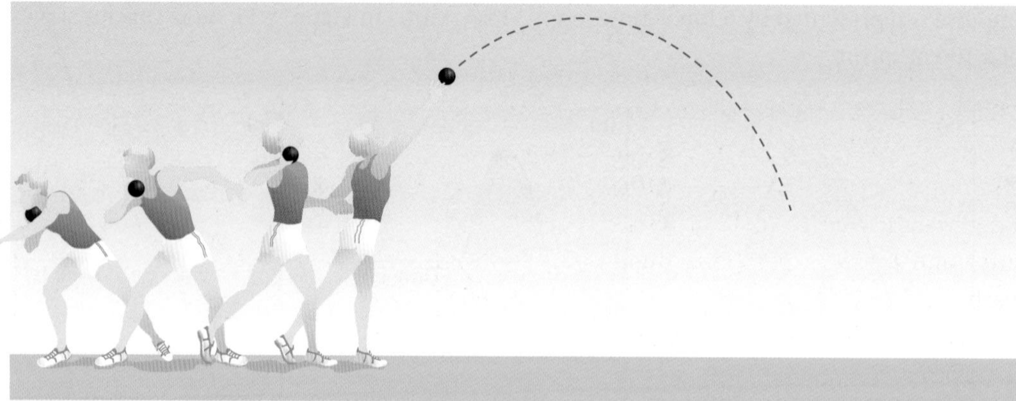
Figure 8.16

If the release height is below the landing height the optimum angle of release is greater than 45°. Shooting in basketball highlights this (assuming the ring is the landing height), as shown in Figure 8.17.

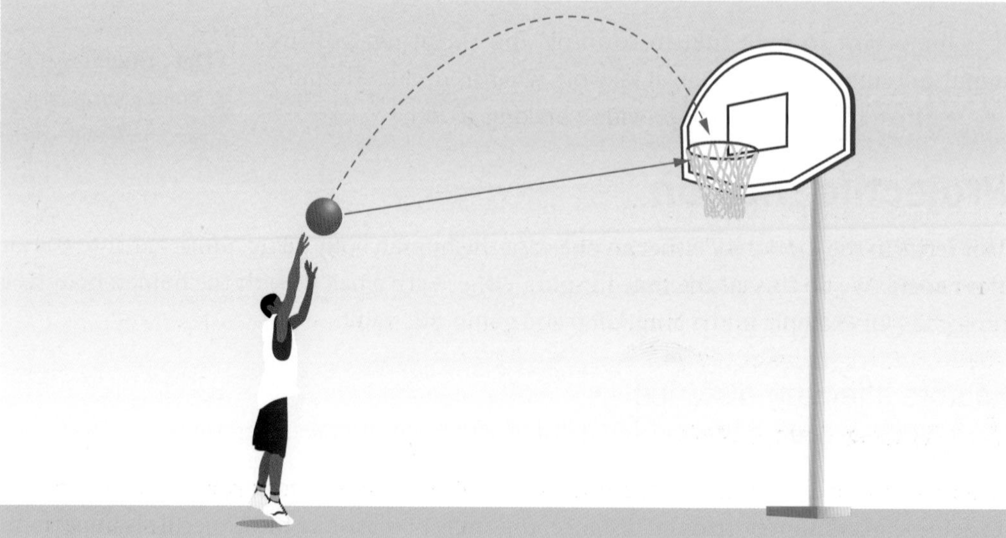
Figure 8.17

Velocity of release

The greater the release velocity of a projectile, the greater the horizontal distance travelled. In the throwing events in athletics, the rotational speed across the circle ensures greater horizontal distance.

Height of release

A greater release height results in an increase in horizontal distance. This means that when fielding a ball in cricket, the taller the fielder the further the distance he can throw the ball, providing the angle of release and velocity of release are the same. In order for a smaller fielder to achieve the same distance, he will have to change the angle or velocity of release.

Forces affecting projectiles

Weight and air resistance are two forces that affect projectiles while they are in the air. Projectiles with a large weight have a small air resistance and follow a parabolic flight path.

Figure 8.18 shows the flight path of a shot put. As the shot has a large mass, the weight arrow is longer than the air resistance arrow. Projectiles with a lighter mass, such as a shuttlecock, are affected by air resistance much more and this causes them to deviate from the parabolic pathway, as shown in Figure 8.19. Compared with the shot, the shuttlecock has a lighter mass and an unusual shape that increases its air resistance. In a serve, the shuttle starts off with a high velocity, provided by the force of the racket. As the shuttle continues its flight path it slows down and the effect of air resistance decreases.

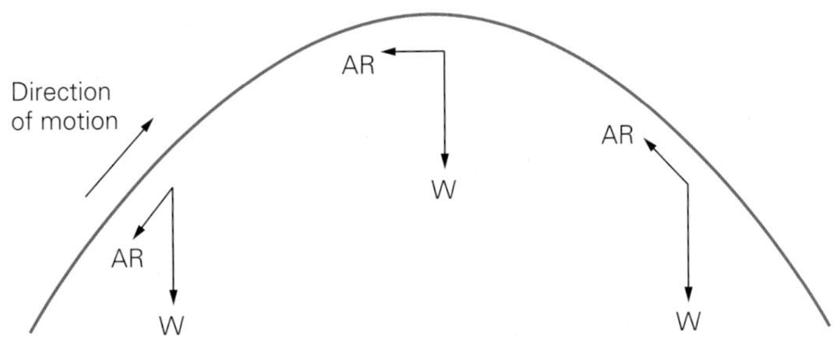

Figure 8.18 The forces acting on the flight path of a shot put

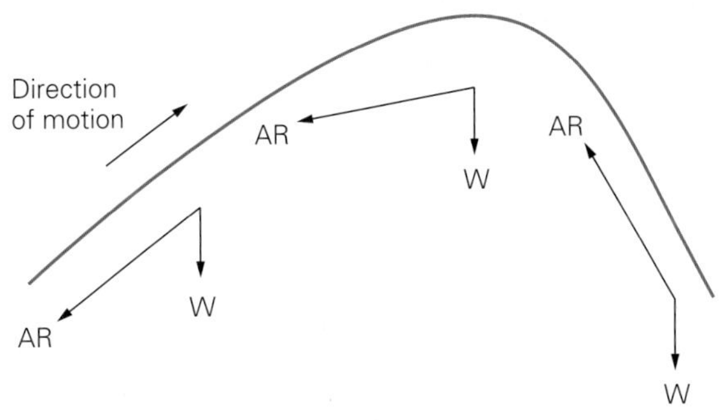

Figure 8.19 The forces acting on the flight path of a shuttlecock

Angular motion

Angular motion is movement around a fixed point or axis — for example, a somersault. Remember, angular motion occurs when a force is applied outside the centre of mass. An off-centre force is referred to as an eccentric force.

Tasks to tackle 8.7

List three sporting examples of a force being applied outside the centre of mass of an object or body to cause rotation.

1 ....

2 ....

3 ....

Axes of rotation

There are three axes of rotation:

- the longitudinal axis, which runs from top to bottom
- the frontal axis, which runs from front to back
- the transverse axis, which runs from side to side across the body

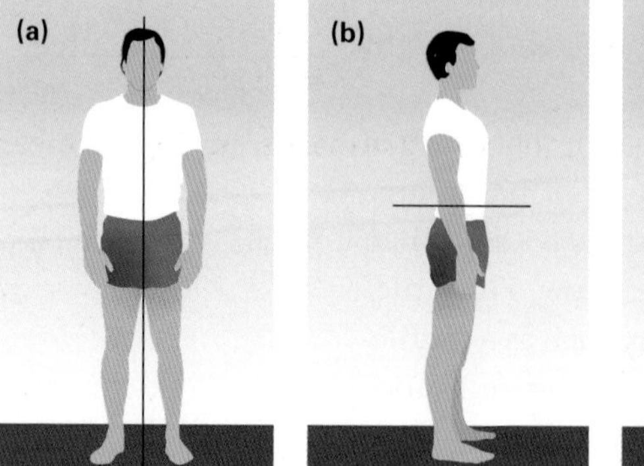

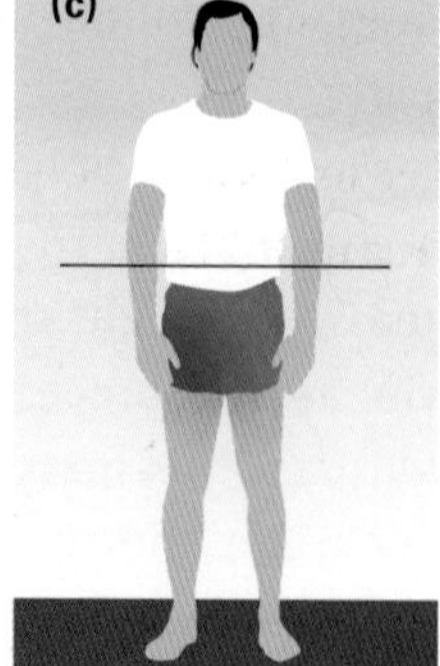

Figure 8.20 (a) The longitudinal axis, (b) the frontal axis and (c) the transverse axis of the human body

Moments of force, or torque

Torque (often called the moment) can be described as a rotational force. It causes an object to turn about its axis of rotation. Increasing the size of the force and the perpendicular distance of the force from the pivotal point (axis of rotation) will increase the moment of the force. Moment of a force or torque can be calculated as follows:

> **Key term**
> **Torque:** a rotational force.

$$\text{moment of force or torque (newton metres)} = \text{force (newtons)} \times \text{perpendicular distance from the fulcrum (metres)}$$

Quantities used in angular motion

Knowledge of the following measurements will be useful in your study of the mechanics of movement:

- **Angular distance** is the angle rotated about an axis when moving from one position to another. Angular distance is measured in radians (1 radian = 57.3 degrees).

- **Angular displacement** is the smallest change in angle between the starting and finishing point. Angular displacement is also measured in radians.
- **Angular speed** is the time it takes to turn through an angle and is measured in radians per second. It is calculated as follows:

$$\text{angular speed (rad s}^{-1}) = \frac{\text{angular distance (rad)}}{\text{time taken (s)}}$$

- **Angular velocity** is a vector quantity as it makes reference to direction. Angular velocity refers to the angular displacement that is covered in a certain time and is calculated as follows:

$$\text{angular velocity (rad s}^{-1}) = \frac{\text{angular displacement (rad)}}{\text{time taken (s)}}$$

- **Angular acceleration** is the rate of change of angular velocity over time. It is calculated as follows:

$$\text{angular acceleration (rad s}^{-2}) = \frac{\text{change in velocity (rad s}^{-1})}{\text{time taken (s)}}$$

Let us look at the example of a gymnast spinning on a bar (Figure 8.21).

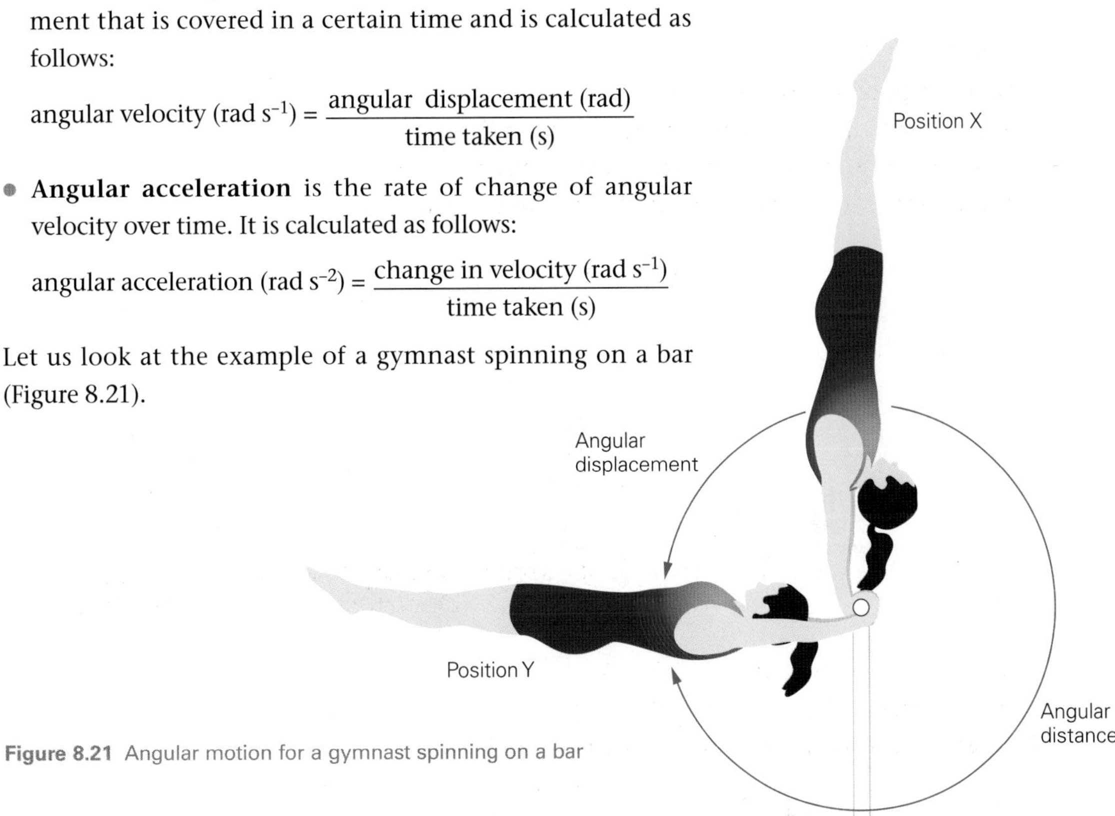

Figure 8.21 Angular motion for a gymnast spinning on a bar

Angular distance	Angular displacement	Angular speed	Angular velocity	Angular acceleration
= 270° = 4.7 radians	= 90° = 1.5 radians	$= \frac{\text{angular distance (rad)}}{\text{time taken (s)}}$ If time taken from position X to position Y = 0.5 s $= \frac{4.7}{0.5}$ $= 9.4 \text{ rad s}^{-1}$	$= \frac{\text{angular displacement (rad)}}{\text{time taken (s)}}$ $= \frac{1.5}{0.5}$ $= 3 \text{ rad s}^{-1}$	$= \frac{\text{change in angular velocity (rad s}^{-1})}{\text{time taken (s)}}$ position X = 0 rad s^{-1} position Y = 3 rad s^{-1} $= \frac{3}{0.5}$ $= 6 \text{ rad s}^{-2}$

Newton's laws of motion related to angular motion

Newton's laws of motion also apply to angular motion (earlier in this chapter we looked at Newton's laws in relation to linear motion). We only need to amend the terminology:

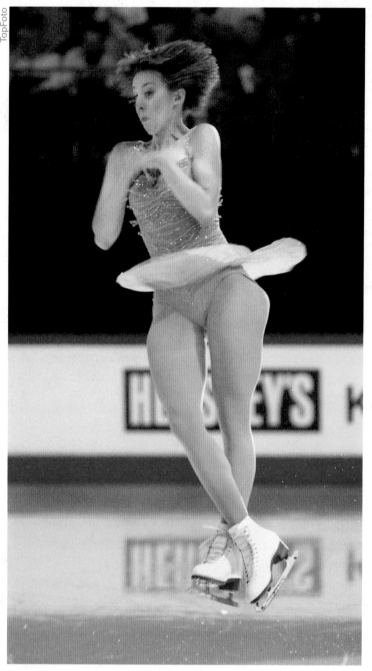

Newton's first law means that the skater will continue to spin until she lands

Newton's first law:
A rotating body will continue in its state of angular motion unless an external force (torque) is exerted upon it.

Think of an ice-skater completing a spinning jump. She will continue to spin until she lands. The ground exerts an external force (torque), which changes her state of angular momentum.

Newton's second law:
The rate of change of angular momentum of a body is proportional to the force (torque) causing it and the change that takes place in the direction in which the force (torque) acts.

For example, leaning forwards from a diving board will create more angular momentum than standing straight.

Newton's third law:
When a force (torque) is applied by one body to another, the second body will exert an equal and opposite force (torque) on the other body.

For example, in a dive, when changing position from a tight tuck to a lay out position, the diver rotates the trunk back (extends the trunk). The reaction is for the lower body to rotate in the opposite direction (extension at the hips).

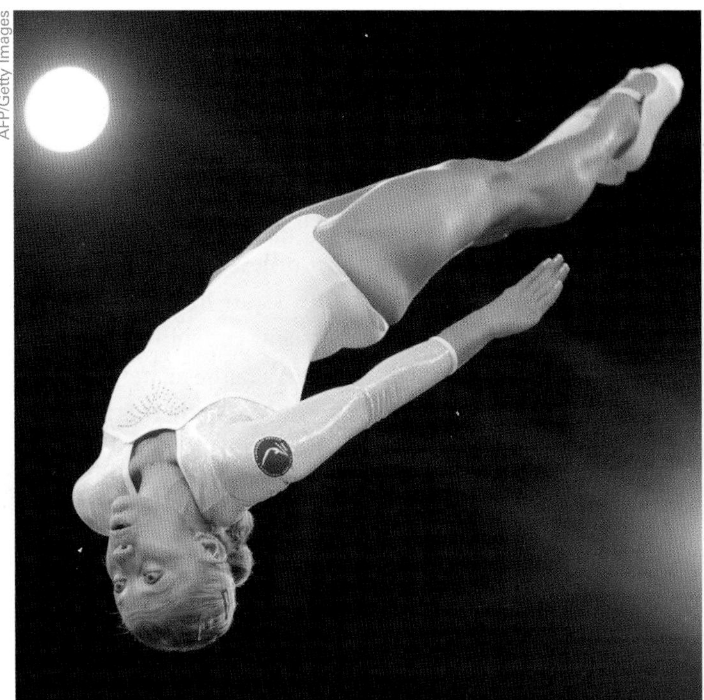
AFP/Getty Images

High moment of inertia

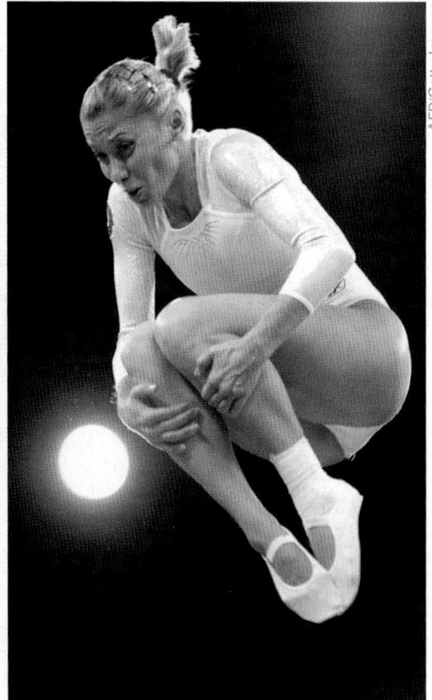
AFP/Getty Images

Low moment of inertia

Moment of inertia

Inertia is a resistance to change in motion, so moment of inertia is the resistance of a body to angular motion (rotation). This depends upon the mass of the body and the distribution of mass around the axis.

Mass of the body/object

The greater the mass, the greater the resistance to change and therefore the greater the moment of inertia. For example, a medicine ball is more difficult to roll along the ground than a tennis ball is.

Distribution of mass from the axis of rotation

The closer the mass is to the axis of rotation, the easier it is to turn — so the moment of inertia is low. Increasing the distance of the distribution of mass from the axis of rotation will increase the moment of inertia. In the example illustrated in the photos, a somersault in a straight position has a higher moment of inertia than the tucked somersault. This is because in the straight position the distribution of the gymnast's mass is further away from the axis of rotation.

Bending (flexion) of the arms and legs reduces the moment of inertia. A pole-vaulter, for example, will flex the knees on the way up to make rotation easier and give him/her more chance of clearing the bar.

Angular momentum

In its simplest form, angular momentum is spin. It involves an object or body in motion around an axis. It depends upon the moment of inertia and angular velocity. These two are inversely proportional — if moment of inertia increases, angular velocity decreases, and vice versa.

Conservation of angular momentum

Angular momentum is a conserved quantity — it stays constant unless an external torque (force) acts upon it (Newton's first law). When an ice-skater executes a spin, for example, there is no change in his angular momentum until he uses his blades to slow the spin down.

The conservation of angular momentum can be highlighted when a figure-skater performs a spin, turning on a longitudinal (vertical) axis. Ice is a friction-free surface so there is no resistance to movement. Only the figure-skater, therefore, can manipulate his moment of inertia to increase or decrease the speed of the spin. At the start of the spin, the arms and leg are stretched out as shown in Figure 8.22. This increases their distance from the axis of rotation, resulting in a large moment of inertia and a large angular momentum in order to start the spin (rotation is slow).

Top tip

Exam questions frequently ask about the control of the speed of rotation. To answer this you need to have knowledge of the relationship between angular momentum and moment of inertia and how this affects the speed of rotation.

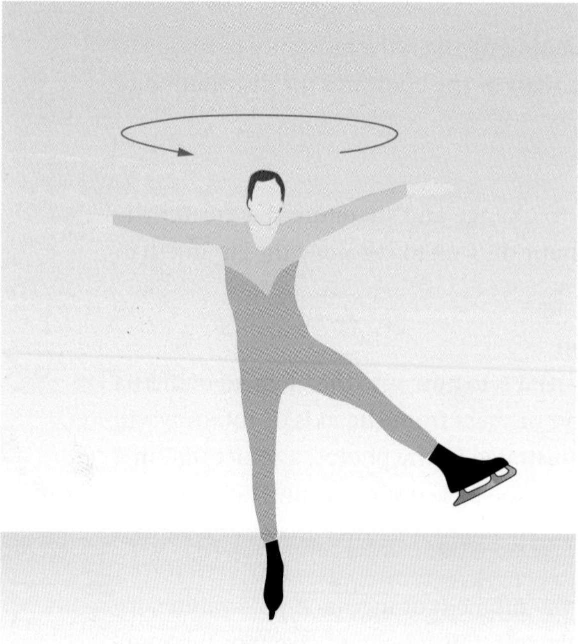

Figure 8.22

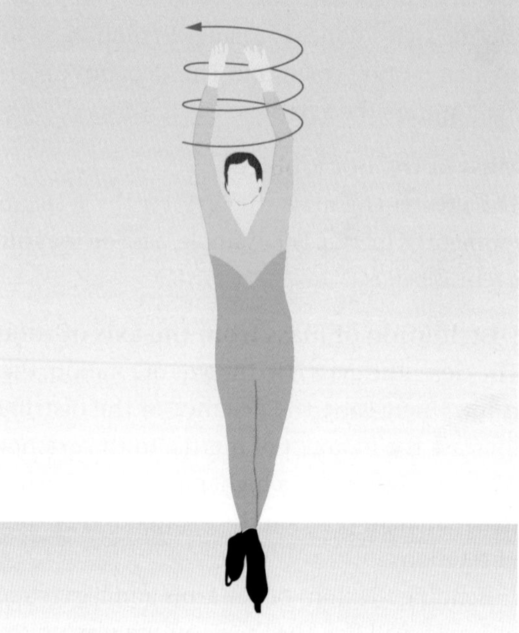

Figure 8.23

When the figure-skater brings his arms and legs back in line with the rest of his body (as in Figure 8.23), the distance of these body parts to the axis of rotation decreases significantly. This reduces the moment of inertia, meaning that angular momentum has to increase. The result is a very fast spin.

Practice makes perfect

1 Use Newton's three laws of motion to explain how a high jumper takes off from the ground. *(6 marks)*

2 Explain, using the idea of vectors, how the leg muscles used in sprinting and high jump produce both maximal horizontal motion and maximal vertical motion. *(5 marks)*

3 What do you understand by the term impulse, and how can an athlete use impulse during sprinting or take-off? *(4 marks)*

4 Explain how an ice-skater is able to alter her speed of rotation by changing her body shape while spinning. *(6 marks)*

Chapter 9

Psychological aspects that optimise performance

Individual influences on the sports performer

What you need to know

By the end of this chapter you should be able to:

- describe the influences on the formation of sporting personalities
- say what attitudes are and how they can be formed and changed
- identify the causes of aggressive behaviour in sport

Personality

Believe it or not, you are unique. Personality is defined as the unique psychological and behavioural characteristics of an individual. In sport, personality affects the way that each individual performer approaches competition. Both Roger Federer and John McEnroe have been successful Wimbledon tennis champions yet have very different personalities (on court at least). Federer is calm and assured, McEnroe was volatile and temperamental. What makes Federer and McEnroe so different? Three major theories outline how a personality develops. These three theories — trait theory, social learning theory and the interactionist approach — are very important because they form the basis not only of personality development, but also of many other topics that you will see in sports psychology.

Trait theory

Trait theory states that we are born with certain personality characteristics, or **traits**, that influence the way in which we behave. These inherited characteristics are fairly stable, in that they stay with us for quite some time. Trait theory therefore suggests that it might be possible to predict the way in which a sports person will behave. For example, an aggressive football player might be prone to commit fouls in a game in which the referee has lost control. It may be a good idea, therefore, if in such a game the coach substituted that player to avoid a sending off. Inherited traits include **extroversion** (being loud and confident) or **introversion** (being shy and quiet). These two opposing traits should be viewed on a sliding scale or continuum since individuals can have a mixture of extroversion and introversion.

> **Key term**
>
> **Trait:** an innate characteristic that could predetermine behaviour.

Personality traits are, at least in part, a function of our biology. The reticular activating system (RAS) regulates the amount of arousal experienced by the brain (see p. 103). Extroverts, whose characteristics include the need to affiliate to other people and social situations, prefer high arousal situations because their RAS operates at comparatively low levels of activity. To this group, high arousal situations are stimulating and enable them to drive towards their goals. Introverts, who do not seek social situations, prefer low arousal conditions because their levels of internal arousal are comparatively high and they do not require the extra external stimuli for drive or motivation.

Other examples of traits include **stability**, which is consistent behaviour, and **instability** which is neurotic behaviour. Again, individuals have a mix of both characteristics but some tend to be more towards one extreme than the other. Figure 9.1 shows how personality can be viewed on a sliding scale.

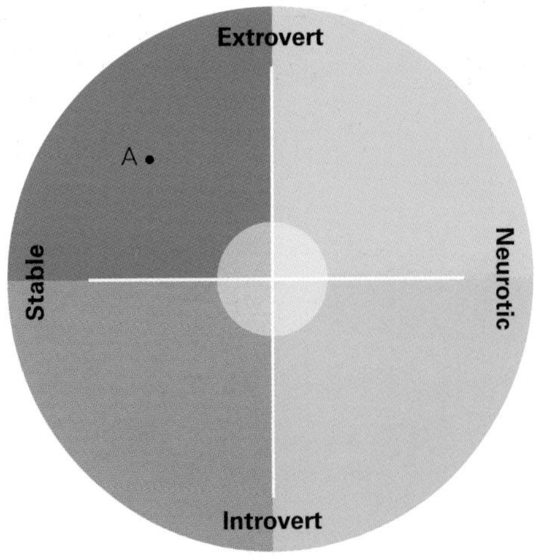

Figure 9.1 A matrix of personality traits — 'stable extrovert' (e.g. point A) describes a personality that is consistently loud and bright

Narrow band

The narrow band approach is a trait theory that groups personality characteristics into two types. **Type A** personalities lack patience and tolerance; they are anxious, but they tend to continue with tasks such as training schedules, even when they feel tired. **Type B** personalities are more relaxed and tolerant and suffer less from anxiety.

Profile of mood states

> **Key term**
> **Profile:** a short description of personal characteristics.

Sports psychologists have attempted to use trait theory to **profile** both successful and unsuccessful sports people. It has been found that successful athletes have certain positive mental characteristics. Morgan investigated performances in different sports and produced a 'profile of mood states' (POMS). In this study, successful athletes scored highly in showing positive moods (vigour) and were low on negative mood states (tension, depression, anger, fatigue, confusion). The less successful athletes showed less vigour but similar profiles for other mood states. A graph that depicts these findings is shown in Figure 9.2. It is often referred to as the 'iceberg profile' since the profile of successful athletes is similar to that of an iceberg when depicted on the graph.

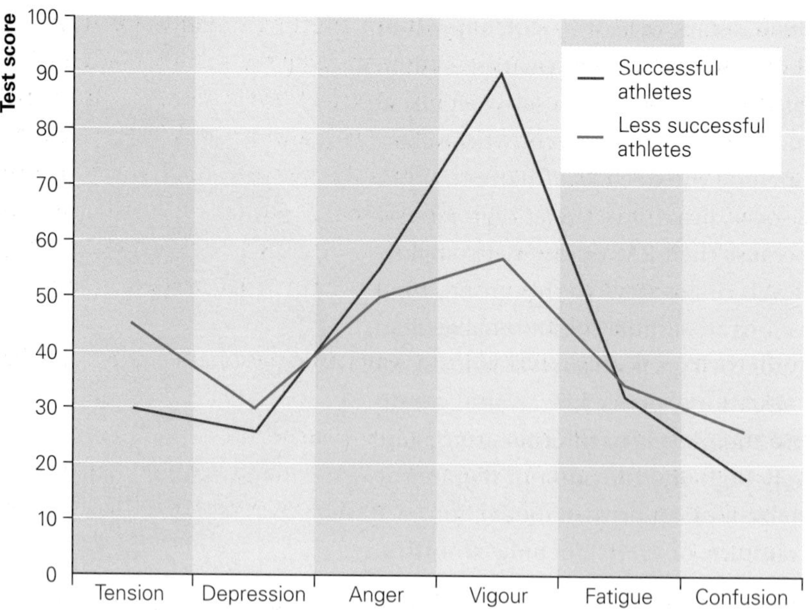

Figure 9.2 Profile of mood states, POMS

Data collection and trait theory

Attempts to profile sporting personalities using trait theory have, however, been largely unsuccessful. In sport, personality can change with the situation. In a game of rugby, for example, a player could be performing with control and clear thinking until they are fouled by an opponent and then their behaviour could change to become aggressive. It is also possible for sporting personalities to behave very differently outside the sporting arena. A boxer may be calm and sociable in his home life yet in the boxing ring he is assertive and highly motivated. It is also true that many of the methods used to measure sporting traits — including questionnaires, observation and physical tests — have rendered the research unreliable, invalid and inconsistent.

Questionnaires can be very quick and yield a lot of information in a short space of time. Examples include the sport competition anxiety test (see Chapter 11). The problem with such questionnaires is that the respondent can fail to understand the question asked or may be tempted to give the answer they feel they ought to give rather than the truth. This can result in a biased response.

Observing behaviour and recording the characteristics of the subject can give a true-to-life picture. However, if the subjects realise that they are being watched, their behaviour can change. This is also a very subjective way of assessing personality characteristics and observers need to be trained so that consistent results can be found. After all, two people watching the same game can have very different opinions on the reasons for success or failure!

Some researchers have suggested that sport can affect personality. For example, physical education builds social qualities, team work and leadership skills. There may be a link between physical exercise and psychological well-being. **Physical testing** for personality includes the measure of heart rate, for example, to assess anxiety and stress. While such measures are factual and objective — so there is valid comparison between results — quite often sports performers do not like to be wired up with assessment equipment while they are playing because it so restrictive to their movement. It has therefore been very difficult to get a true measure of anxiety during a real-life game, such as a cup final, and most results have been recorded during training situations.

Therefore, in terms of the reliability of the research into personality traits, it can be said that the results may:

- lack consistency (for example, due to subjective observation)
- lack internal validity (for example, due to untruthful questionnaire results)
- lack external validity (for example, when physical testing environments do not match the wider sporting environment)

Trait theory is therefore a poor predictor of behaviour and it can be argued that the need to take account of personality *change* is more important. Social learning theory tries to address this problem.

Tasks to tackle 9.1

The following table shows the main methods of collecting information on personality. Copy and complete the table by suggesting at least one advantage and one disadvantage for each method in the appropriate column.

Method	Advantages	Disadvantages
Questionnaire		
Observation		
Physiological		

Social learning theory

Social learning theory argues that instead of remaining stable, personality characteristics develop over time. Individuals learn from sporting situations and other experiences (the environment), and copy other people who are held in high esteem. Such people are known as

> **Key terms**
>
> **Significant others:** people we hold in high esteem.
>
> **Socialisation:** the process of associating with others and accepting their behaviour as the norm.

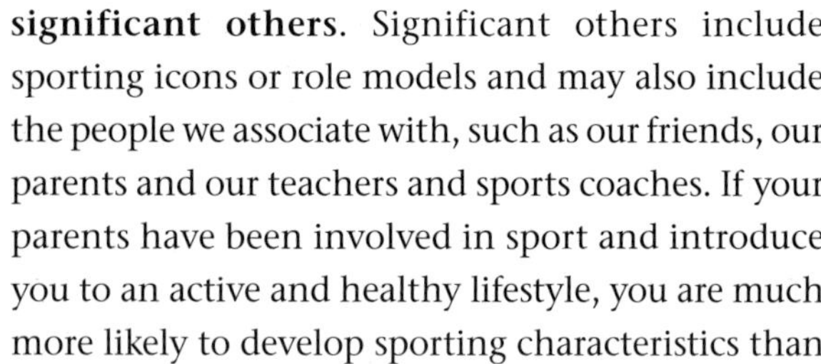

significant others. Significant others include sporting icons or role models and may also include the people we associate with, such as our friends, our parents and our teachers and sports coaches. If your parents have been involved in sport and introduce you to an active and healthy lifestyle, you are much more likely to develop sporting characteristics than if you had not been exposed to such competitive situations. Think of some of the parent and child combinations that have featured in professional sport. For example, the former county cricketer and Leeds rugby player Liam Botham is the son of Sir Ian Botham, who played cricket for England.

We learn personality characteristics by a process called **socialisation**. We associate with significant others and begin to accept and display their behaviour. For example, if a group of friends all play in the same junior football team then it is a good bet that during break at school, the same friends will end up playing football together in the playground. The social learning process often follows the pattern:

observe → identify → reinforce → copy

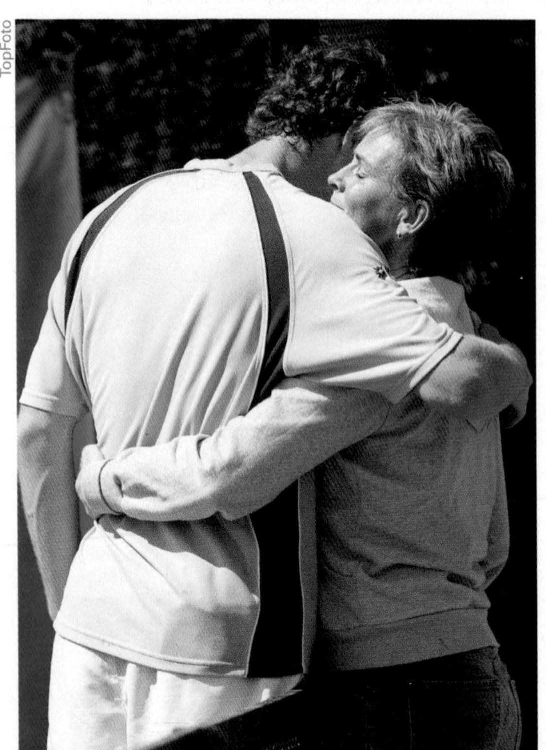

TopFoto

Judy Murray, mother of Britain's tennis number one Andy Murray, is a leading tennis coach

In other words, we see behaviour, realise what it is and if it is successful we will try it ourselves. Individuals are likely to copy behaviour that fits in with their own age, gender, ability and values. Behaviour tends to be copied if is high profile, powerful, consistent, successful and reinforced. For example, the goal scoring celebrations of professional football players that are highlighted in the media are often copied by youngsters because of the high status value of the football role model to the youngster.

The interactionist approach

The interactionist approach encompasses the best of both worlds by combining the features of trait theory and social learning theory. It suggests that an individual's behaviour is a result of both personality *and* the influence of the environment. This is summed up by the formula:

$$B = f(P \times E)$$

This means that behaviour (*B*) is a function (f) of personality trait (*P*) and environmental situation (*E*). In other words, people are born with stable personality characteristics, but these characteristics are then adapted to suit the situation. For example, a hockey captain may act as a calming influence to settle the team's nerves before a big game, but in the closing stages of that game if the team is a goal down the same captain may use all her powers of motivation to drive the team on to score the equalising goal. This theory accounts for changes in behaviour and is perhaps more applicable to modern-day sport because it takes into account how behaviour can change during a game.

Top tip

Exam questions, particularly longer ones, may ask you to discuss all of the psychological theories dealt with in this chapter. Make sure that you give all of the conflicting views, and note that it is the interactionist approach that students tend to forget.

Achievement motivation

Achievement motivation is a concept of personality that looks at how individual athletes approach a competitive situation. Some players welcome the challenge and feel very confident as they approach a big game or are asked to do a demanding task. Some do not welcome competition and will be tempted to leave to others those tasks that present a risk of failure. Those who welcome competition and seek out a challenge are said to be motivated by the 'need to achieve', and display **NACH characteristics**. Those who avoid competition and are not willing to accept a challenge are said to display the 'need to avoid failure', or **NAF characteristics**.

The features of a NACH personality are as follows:

- The athlete is very competitive and welcomes a challenge.
- Risks are taken, even if there is a chance of failure.
- The performer is keen to see feedback on the outcome.
- Confidence is displayed.
- Personal responsibility is taken for the result.
- The athlete blames internal reasons, such as his/her ability, for success.

The features of a NAF personality are as follows:

- Challenge is avoided and the athlete may seek easy targets.
- Lack of confidence may be present.
- Feedback is unwelcome.
- External reasons are blamed for lack of success.

The adoption of these NACH or NAF characteristics can depend not only on the performer, but also on the situation. Sometimes an athlete feels confident and prepared to have a go while at other times he/she may prefer to leave the challenge to someone else.

Naturally confident personalities — those said to display trait confidence — will be likely to show a competitive approach. Those who have had experience in a similar situation before, especially if they have succeeded, will also be likely to show NACH characteristics. A young performer at school, for example, might relish the chance to show his classmates the advanced gymnastic skills that he has developed already at gym club.

One of the most important influences on the adoption of a NACH or NAF approach concerns how much the task means to the individual. In other words, what is the incentive? A task that can be achieved easily offers little incentive for the performer and no sense of satisfaction when it is completed. A task that is hard to achieve, one where failure is possible, offers much more personal incentive and a sense of achievement when completed. Imagine going mountain walking and finding two routes you can take: an easy stroll that you are guaranteed to finish, and a hard three peaks challenge that not everyone completes. Which one would you do? Which offers the greatest incentive? The harder route is taken by those who have a need to achieve and who wish to gain satisfaction from completing the task.

Coaches want their players to maintain a competitive approach and to show the need to keep on achieving. To help maintain motivation, the coach should set targets that can be achieved in the early coaching sessions and then make these targets more difficult as the players improve. Any success achieved by the players should be rewarded with praise and positive feedback and the players should be made to feel that they are responsible for any success achieved. The coach could point out role models who have similar ability to their own players and who have achieved success. The challenges faced by the players should be hard enough to offer an incentive but not so impossible to achieve that confidence is lost. In such a way, motivation to compete can be maintained.

Attitudes

An attitude is the way a person views something or tends to behave towards it. You may have heard someone described as having a bad attitude in class, for example because he/she does not like doing written work. In sport, both negative and positive attitudes exist and there are a number of ways that such attitudes are formed.

An attitude is made up of three parts, referred to as the triadic model:

- The **cognitive component** relates to what we think or believe. In sport, the cognitive part of attitude is shown by a belief in the benefits of exercise, for example the knowledge that going to the gym is healthy.
- The **affective component** relates to feelings and emotions. For example, when we go to the gym we may enjoy it and show enthusiasm towards our training.
- The **behavioural component** relates to what we do and how we behave. For example, going to the gym three times a week is an indication of a positive behavioural attitude towards exercise.

Tasks to tackle 9.2

Give an example from sport that shows each of the three components of an attitude. You can use examples from your own experience if you wish to show how you may have shown a cognitive attitude, an affective interpretation and a behavioural response.

Key terms

Cognitive: describes a thought process or belief.

Affective: describes an emotional feeling or interpretation.

Behavioural: describes an action — a physical response to a situation.

Forming attitudes

There is a link between all three parts of an attitude. However, the cognitive component (what we think) it not always reflected in the behavioural component (what we do). If you posed the question 'Is going to the gym good for your health?' most people would answer 'Yes'. But not all those people would actually go to the gym on a regular basis. They would use the affective part of the attitude to justify their actions: 'I don't go to the gym because I do other forms of exercise like walking the dog and I like the fresh air.' It is the affective, or emotional, part of the attitude that often determines our actions. Attitudes, therefore, do not always predict behaviour, although they can predict specific responses to attitude objects if all three components of the attitude are similar. Other influences, such as personality traits, may also mean that attitudes alone are not a good means of predicting behaviour.

Attitudes are formed from an individual's beliefs, influences and experiences — they are learned responses. It is important to note that such influences can be either positive or negative, and so attitudes can also be either positive or negative.

We have already seen how people held in high esteem, in other words significant others, are a major influence on an individual's beliefs and attitudes. Significant others include parents and friends, teachers and sports coaches and, very importantly, role models that we may look up to. Such role models do not necessarily have to be elite performers at the top professional level (sometimes we may feel that we will not be able to match such talent); they may be people of our own age who have worked hard to reach a good level of performance or who simply enjoy taking part. A youngster with sporty parents, who has been encouraged to take up a sport by being taken to early coaching sessions, may begin to enjoy the activity and develop positive attitudes. On the other hand, a child whose parents are not sporty and who refuse to get involved in sport may not develop positive attitudes to any sporting activity.

Individuals' past experiences may influence their future attitudes. If, for example, we attended a gymnastics class as a youngster and stretched too far, causing an injury, we may have developed negative attitudes to gymnastics. If we went to the class and enjoyed it, we may have developed positive attitudes towards gymnastics.

The media have a powerful influence on the development of sporting attitudes. When the England cricket team won the Ashes against Australia in 2006, the sport enjoyed far more extensive and enthusiastic media coverage than usual. The media hype surrounding that win led to very positive approaches towards cricket and a lot of young players were attracted to the sport. A few months later, in early 2007, the same cricket team went to Australia, lost the series after a spate of poor performances, and were subsequently 'slated' by the press. Negative attitudes towards the team began to develop and the positive thoughts regarding cricket became more negative. This may have contributed to the fact that no terrestrial channel bid for coverage of live test cricket when the rights were redistributed in mid-2008.

Such a turn around in attitudes in such a short space of time suggests that attitudes can be readily changed. From a coaching point of view, it is desirable to change negative attitudes into positive ones.

Changing attitudes

One way to change an attitude is to use the simple technique of persuasion. Persuasion is most effective when it is carried out by an expert. For example, persuading someone that it might be a good idea to go to a fitness class, despite their reservations, might be easier if the advice came from a fitness conditioner or health expert.

Another way to change a negative attitude into a positive one is to use the concept of **cognitive dissonance**. This is a process that challenges existing beliefs. Imagine a rugby prop forward being told that as part of his training he has to take part in some aerobics. The prop may believe that aerobics is for girls and refuse to take part. The coach could challenge this cognitive part of the attitude by suggesting that aerobics is a good measure of stamina and only the fittest people can maintain a constant work rate for a full hour. In response to the challenge the prop may then go and do his aerobics session.

Other ways in which negative attitudes can be changed include making the training sessions fun and enjoyable, with variety in practice, so that the affective part of the attitude is developed in a positive way. Giving young players early success will help them to develop a belief in their ability and foster a positive approach. For example, young tennis players play a half court version of the game with a sponge ball to allow early success and enjoyment. The use of rewards and plenty of positive reinforcement will help to promote confidence and enjoyment. The cognitive part of the attitude could be developed by simply pointing out the benefits of exercise to the performer.

> **Top tip**
>
> Questions on attitudes often ask for the ways in which attitudes are formed. Remember that the influences on the formation of attitudes can be positive or negative. For example, a role model can be a positive sporting icon who demonstrates fair play, but role models can also be negative and promote hostile behaviour.

Sometimes attitudes can become very strong and an expectation develops. Extreme attitudes can develop into a prejudice — a generalising assumption that may not be correct. Undesirable and prejudicial attitudes can be formed on the basis of race, gender, age or physical ability, and even against sporting officials.

Imagine that your favourite football team is playing in a cup semi-final. The referee

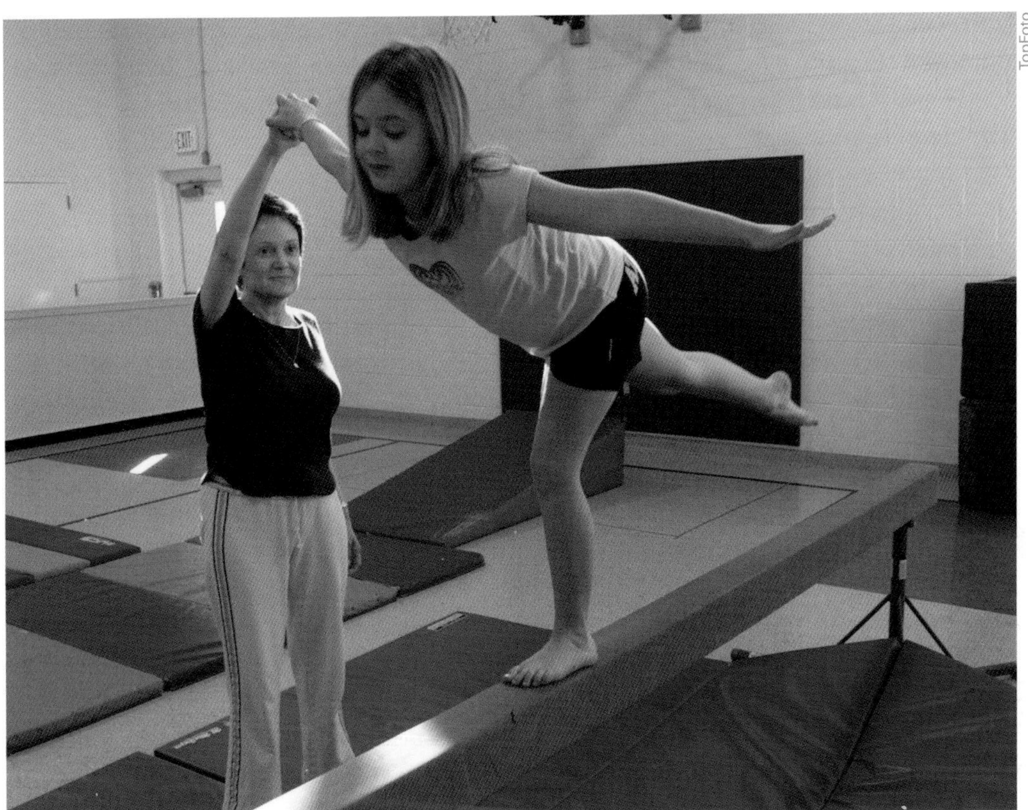

TopFoto

Successful coaching offers youngsters the possibility of early success to promote positive attitudes

gives the opposition a penalty when it is clearly shown in television replays and in newspaper photographs that the foul was committed outside the penalty box. The opponents score from the spot kick and your team is out of the competition. A few weeks later, the same referee is due to officiate at your team's next home game. As he runs out onto the field he is greeted by a chorus of boos from the home fans. In fact, every referee who has taken charge of home games has been ridiculed in the last few weeks by the home fans. All referees are bad, aren't they? In this example, a prejudice against match officials has been formed on the basis of one bad experience. The referee perhaps had a good game apart from that one error, but the influence of the media has focused attention on the official. When the home crowd starts to boo the referee, everyone seems to join in, perhaps because of a need to fit in with the crowd and not be left out.

The above example shows how a prejudice can be formed from a past experience, by the influence of the media and by fitting in with the norm of group behaviour. Historical influences and cultural differences can also be responsible for the formation of a prejudice. Few England football fans think positively of the Argentine player Diego Maradonna since his infamous 'hand of God' goal that knocked England out of the World Cup in 1986, even though it was a long time ago and he was a great player.

To counter a prejudice, coaches use some of the methods involved in promoting positive attitudes. Persuasion by an expert or the use of cognitive dissonance will help to change a prejudicial view. A coach can also prevent a prejudice from developing by reinforcing fair play in training and punishing behaviour that may be seen as being unfairly biased. Most professional sports have a fair play charter by which any racist or sexist comments result in a ban from playing or watching the sport. The media can further prevent prejudice by highlighting the positive aspects of fair play and equality that frequently happen in sport. The coach can point out positive role models who play the game in a fair and balanced fashion.

Attitudes — since they are specifically directed at attitude objects — can theoretically be used to predict behaviour. It may be possible to predict how someone with a negative attitude will behave in a specific situation. For example, a jockey may not be expected to try his best in a game of rugby. Yet behaviour is unpredictable, and the jockey might do his best in the rugby session just to show what he is capable of. We should note that the cognitive part of the attitude does not always reflect how we behave and therefore using attitudes to predict behaviour is not always reliable.

Attitudes can be measured by questionnaires in a similar way to personality (see p. 68). Attitudes are measured on 'attitude scales', such as the Likert scale, on which the subject has to state the extent to which he/she agrees or disagrees with a statement. Attitudes can also be measured by observation of behaviour.

Attitudes are very important in sports performance because they affect effort and motivation. Promoting positive attitudes is a way of encouraging participation in sport.

Aggression in sport

While watching a game on television you may have heard the commentator describe one of the players as being very 'aggressive' when making a hard tackle. If the player concerned was trying to win the ball and played within the rules, then the tackle was not actually aggressive, it was assertive. **Aggression** is defined as an intent to harm. An aggressive act is outside the rules of the game and is often prompted by reactive behaviour that is out of control. For example, a rugby player who is pulled back when chasing a kick might react by punching the offender. **Assertion** is within the rules of the game and is well-motivated behaviour that is more in control, such as a hard yet fair tackle during a game of rugby.

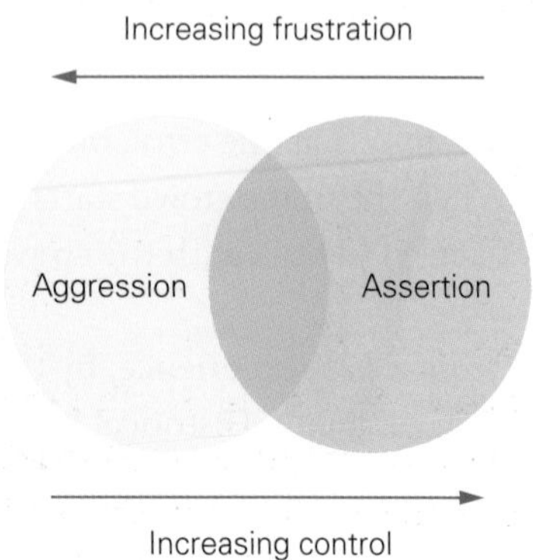

Figure 9.3 Aggression and assertion

There is an overlap between the definitions of aggression and assertion as shown in Figure 9.3. In the example of the rugby tackle above, there may be fair contact but there may also be intent to make sure the ball carrier feels the impact.

Hostile aggression is a specific intent to harm another person. Sometimes the aggression shown in sport can be very hostile, for example when a reaction to a foul is designed to inflict injury on another player. **Instrumental aggression** is less personal and lacks the intent to injure someone else but it is aimed at breaking the rules or abusing the equipment, for example a tennis player shouting at an umpire to dispute a line call.

Key terms

Hostile aggression: an intent to harm; a reaction to mounting anger and frustration.

Instrumental aggression: no specific intent to harm another person, but a purposeful action aimed at breaking the rules or abusing equipment.

Tasks to tackle 9.3

There is some overlap between the definitions of aggression and assertion. Use your knowledge of aggression in sport to construct your own diagram, Powerpoint or Word document to show some of the main features of an aspect of aggression. Use this example to help you.

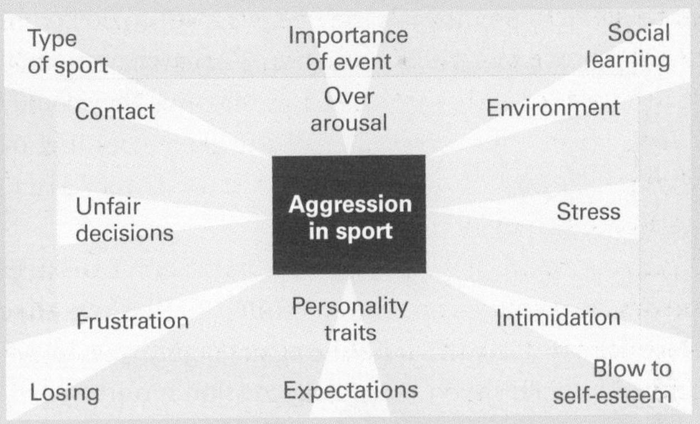

There are four theories that explain why aggression happens in sport.

Instinct theory

This theory states that we are all born with an aggressive instinct that will surface under provocation or threat. The nature of this theory lies in evolution, which teaches that humans once had to be naturally aggressive hunters and defenders of territory. The aggressive instinct can be manifested on the pitch when defending a goal or reacting to a foul, for example. Some players only need slight provocation to react in a violent manner, while others need much more intimidation before losing their cool.

Frustration–aggression theory

Aggression can be caused in sport by the frustration of being prevented from achieving what we want to achieve. For example, an ice-hockey player prevented from reaching the puck by a defender's illegal use of the stick might take out his frustration on the defender by lashing out. This tendency to react aggressively when our goals are blocked is called the frustration–aggression hypothesis, or F–A hypothesis. The F–A hypothesis suggests that aggression is inevitable once an individual is stopped from achieving his/her aim, and aggression will immediately develop in response to the mounting frustration. The hypothesis also states that if the individual can let this aggression out, perhaps by retaliation, then the

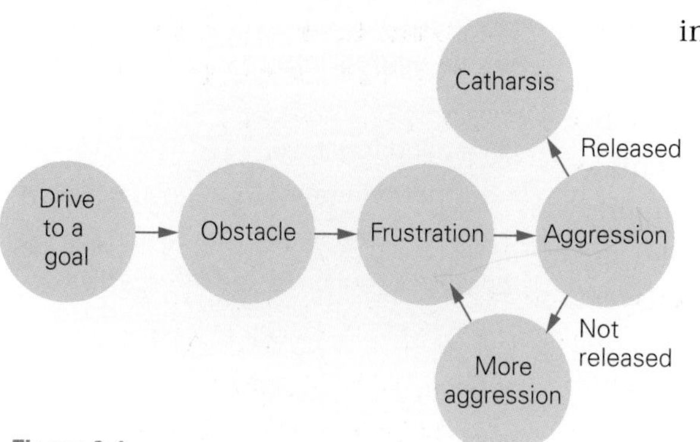

Figure 9.4
The frustration–aggression hypothesis

Key term

Catharsis: a reduction in frustration or anger as a result of releasing aggressive inclinations or 'letting go'.

Top tip

A nature versus nurture debate runs through the personality, aggression and attitude theories. The nature approach, exemplified by the instinct theory of aggression and the trait theory of personality, supports the view that behaviour is innate, consistent and predictable. The nurture approach is based on social learning theory, and suggests that behaviour is learned from significant others and from our experiences, especially if such experiences are reinforced. The interactionist view combines the nature and nurture approaches by suggesting that behavioural change is a result of differing situations. You may find it helpful to group the theories into nature and nurture when answering exam questions.

inclination to be aggressive will be reduced. If, however, the player is unable to get rid of his/her frustration, then the aggression will become more intense and lead to even more frustration and subsequent aggression.

The release of aggression is called **catharsis**, literally meaning 'cleansing the emotions'. It is common to see players in a game get wound up and indulge in pushing and shoving, only to calm down once their little spat is over. If those players were unable to indulge in the pushing and shoving, they could harbour the aggression for the rest of the game. Holding on to the aggressive inclination is seen in this theory as a form of punishment.

Aggressive cue theory

While the first two theories of aggression suggest some natural aggressive inclination, the next two suggest that aggression is nurtured.

The aggressive cue hypothesis proposes that aggression occurs as a result of a learned cue or trigger. This trigger could be something that has developed in the past. A player who has an existing rivalry with a particular opponent, for example, will perhaps only reach certain levels of aggression when confronted by that rival, who acts as the cue. The cue could be self-activated. Think of a boxer grinding one fist into the other glove as though in anticipation of making contact with the opponent. Alternatively, the cue can be learned from, and sometimes activated by, the coach. In boxing, coaches at the ring-side can be seen urging their athletes to direct their aggression towards the target — in this case, the coach acts as the cue.

Social learning theory

Aggression can also be nurtured by learning from other people — social learning. In the same way that personality traits are in part learned from significant others, such as friends and our peers, then aggressive acts can be copied from sporting role models and fellow players. Aggression will be copied especially if the aggressive act is successfully reinforced. In a game of basketball, if the captain fouls an opponent and the foul prevents the opponent from scoring, other players may be tempted to copy this unacceptable behaviour in order to win the game. Aggressive acts are more likely to be copied if they are consistent, performed by someone of our own age and if they are powerful.

Controlling aggression

Aggression is not desirable in sport because it can cause injury, and because players who are aggressive tend to be stressed and unable to perform at their best. Coaches and players therefore have a responsibility to reduce aggression. This can be done in a number of ways.

The coach could substitute players who behave aggressively on the pitch, or punish players with fines if they get sent off. In training, aggressive acts should be criticised and non-aggressive acts should be encouraged with praise. The coach could introduce cognitive techniques, such as imagery and mental rehearsal (see Chapter 11), to lower arousal and stress, and the responsibility of the player to the team should be emphasised by pointing out that giving away penalties for foul play is letting the team down.

Players should learn to walk away from aggressive situations and calm down by focusing on the game and not on retaliation. Players could **channel** their aggressive response into more assertive behaviour, and use physical relaxation techniques before high-pressure games to make sure they stay in control. Players can also help each other to avoid the consequences of aggression by using peer group pressure — in other words, they could remind each other not to get involved in irresponsible, aggressive acts.

> Key term
>
> **Channelling:** re-directing the drive caused by increased frustration into an assertive, rather than an aggressive, response.

The referee can play an important role in reducing aggression by applying the rules in a consistent and fair manner so that frustrations are reduced. The referee should punish acts of aggression so that standards are set for fair play and any sanctions handed out by the referee should be immediate. The referee could prevent aggression by simply talking to players to calm them down before they commit a foul.

Practice makes perfect

1. The performance and behaviour of a sports performer may be affected by his/her personality. What is the trait theory of personality? *(3 marks)*
2. Some performers show a negative attitude to training and playing. How could a negative attitude be changed into a positive one in sport? *(4 marks)*
3. Aggression is an unwelcome feature of sports performance. What can a coach or player do to reduce the aggressive tendencies that sport can sometimes generate? *(4 marks)*

Chapter 10 Psychological aspects that optimise performance

Playing in a team

What you need to know

By the end of this chapter you should be able to:

- understand the dynamics of group performance
- define the factors that affect group performance
- understand how the role of the leader is important in helping the team

Team dynamics

A group is a collection of individuals who work together to achieve a common goal. In sporting terms this could mean your hockey team, which trains and plays together each week in the hope of winning the league. According to Steiner, the success that such a team achieves is based on the following formula:

actual productivity = potential productivity – faulty processes

Actual productivity refers to the result; potential productivity is the best performance the team could achieve if everything went just right; and the faulty processes are the factors that make things go wrong. In other words, the 1–0 win in our last league game (actual productivity) is based on our best possible performance (potential productivity) minus all the things that went wrong during the game (faulty processes).

The potential of the group could be improved by simply having the best players, but the coach should remember that it is how such players interact and work together that produces the best results. Some teams get fantastic results with average players who give their best and work for each other, while other teams have great players but do not always win. Faulty processes affecting a team include coordination problems, lack of cohesion and lack of motivation from some team members.

Top tip

Learn your definitions. Many short exam questions will ask for the meaning of such terms as potential productivity and actual productivity.

Key terms

Actual productivity: the result; the level of attainment on the task.

Potential productivity: the group's best possible performance, influenced by interaction and player quality.

Faulty processes: the factors that reduce group potential, such as poor coordination, social loafing (page 84) and the Ringlemann effect (page 84).

Stages in group formation

According to the psychologist Carron, a group or team is formed over time by passing through four stages, sometimes known as antecedants:

- The **forming stage** — members of the group develop an affinity with each other based on their desire to share a common goal. In sport this could happen, for example, at the first training session undertaken by a group of players who are hoping to be selected for the college rugby team. After the first training session, the players might begin to socialise with each other when they meet in the college recreation area and a bond between them begins to form.
- The **storming stage** — differences of opinion and conflicts within the group may begin to surface. In the college rugby team example, it may emerge that two players are trying to get into the team in the same position and a rivalry develops between them.
- The **norming stage** — the group or team members begin to resolve their differences and settle down into a team with long-term potential. The two players trying out for the same position might solve the problem by agreeing that one of them should play in a different role, a role with which they are now familiar.
- The **performing stage** — finally, the team begins to fulfil its potential and concentrate on achieving its goals. Regular fixtures are fulfilled and the team members enjoy playing their chosen sport.

Tasks to tackle 10.1

The four stages of group formation are forming, storming, norming and performing. Imagine that you are about to join a local hockey team. Describe the characteristics of each of the four stages of formation that you may experience from when you first join the team.

Cohesion and coordination within the team

Coordination problems — seemingly small issues relating to timing and effective communication — can have a significant impact on sports performance. A defender who fails to communicate effectively with fellow defenders might end up leaving an attacker free and giving away a goal. Poor tactics and strategies also result in coordination problems. For example, the players in a basketball team might be instructed to use a one-on-one defence when the individual speed of some of the opponents means it would be better to operate in a zone.

Coordination problems within the team affect group cohesion. **Cohesion** is defined as the degree to which members of a team unite to achieve a common goal. There are two types of cohesion:

- **Task cohesion** involves the group members working together to achieve a goal.
- **Social cohesion** is about how individual team members get on.

Key terms

Interaction: working together to achieve a goal.

Coordination: work and effort that is timed and matched to produce success.

Cohesion: the degree to which members of a team unite to achieve a common goal.

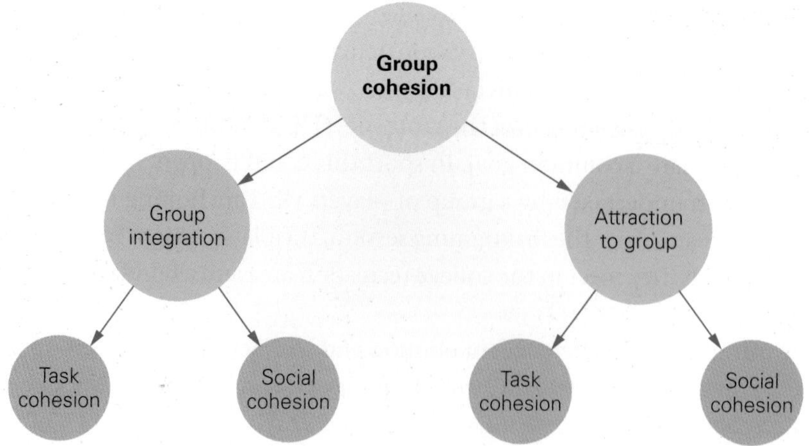

Figure 10.1 The task and social cohesion of individuals combine to give group cohesion

Top tip

More advanced exam questions might ask you to account for the influence of task cohesion *and* social cohesion on team success, so make sure you can describe the importance of both. Remember that task cohesion alone can produce results, but is best accompanied by social cohesion.

Tasks to tackle 10.2

Make a list of the factors that you think could affect team cohesion. For each factor that you identify, state whether you think it affects task cohesion, social cohesion or both. For example, the personality of the players in the team is a factor that could influence social cohesion.

Generally, the best results are achieved when both task cohesion and social cohesion occur, and there is little doubt that successful teams show a high degree of cohesion. Nevertheless, even if some members of the team do not get on socially, they can still produce excellent results with task cohesion alone. Personal differences can be put aside in order to achieve results. Social cohesion does, however, help to promote group interaction.

Both types of cohesion are involved in attraction to a group, and integration within it. Figure 10.1 shows how a player could be attracted to a team for social reasons, to meet and work with others, and for achievement reasons — they like working as a team and think this team will be successful. Once in the group, the player has to integrate with other team members to get the task done — a defensive player needs to communicate with fellow defenders to make sure no goals are conceded, for example.

Influences on cohesion

There are a number of factors that affect both group cohesion and coordination. These factors may be seen as the forces acting on the group that keep the group together.

The type of sport is important in this regard. Sports such as marathon running depend on the individual

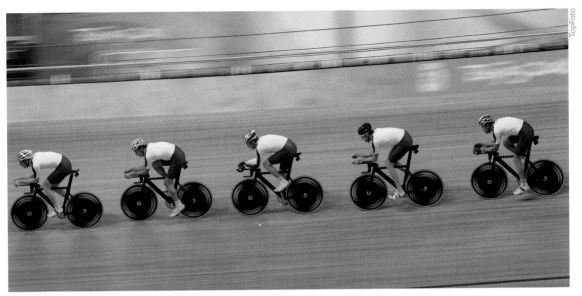
TopFoto

Some sports require high levels of coordination to avoid both failure and injury

athlete and do not need much coordination with others. Team sports such as netball, on the other hand, require a high degree of coordination and cooperation and the interaction of team members is important. There is also more potential for things to go wrong in a team because it is more likely that someone will make a mistake. Sports that are performed in a pair, such as tennis doubles, require interaction and cohesion. Think how vital it is for a double sculls rowing pair to get their mutual timing right. Timing is also important in team coordination. When a set move is performed in rugby it is important that all the players time their runs to perfection.

The personalities of the players also influence cohesion. It is important that the members of the team get on socially and that their personalities 'gel'. Imagine a group of extroverts all vying for attention within the group — a mix of both loud and quiet personalities is better for group harmony.

The rewards on offer can affect team morale and motivation. The desire to win a major cup game will tend to bind the team together in the drive for success. Personal differences are often forgotten in order to achieve success. In other words, the cohesion related to the task is stronger than the cohesion related to social aspects.

Cohesion and coordination are also affected by past success and the probability of future success. If a team has already beaten a particular opponent in the cup, then the players may well look forward with confidence to playing the same opponent again in the league — the good chance of a win will bring a desire to play.

Leadership can also affect team coordination. The captain should encourage and reward the team, with player of the match incentives for example.

Social loafing

A lack of effort by individual team members is called **social loafing**. This can have an effect on team cohesion and performance because it reduces the motivation in the team as a whole. Social loafing can occur when:

- an individual player feels that his/her efforts are not being recognised. This is known as a lack of performance identification. Players might give up if they think that their efforts will not change the result. If the team is losing 5–0 with only a couple of minutes to go there might be no point in trying.
- there is no reward on offer, such as a player of the match award. If the players lack confidence or motivation they might be more prepared to leave it to others to do all the work.
- the players perceive that others are not trying. They might think 'If she isn't putting any effort in, why should I?'
- the team captain is a poor leader and fails to encourage the team
- there is a perceived lack of ability. If a player feels that he/she is not as good as some others in the team, there may be a tendency to leave the majority of the work to the better players.

Social loafing is not desirable within a team so the coach should employ tactics to reduce its effect. The best way to prevent social loafing is to highlight individual performance and one of the best ways to achieve this is to use statistics. The number of tackles, the number of assists and the success rate of shots are all examples of data that players can be given after the game to provide feedback and show that they have been noticed. The coach should also make sure that players are encouraged and motivated during the game and that suitable rewards are on offer. Most clubs have a player of the year award to maintain motivation throughout the season. Confidence could be raised by pointing out the contribution players have made to the result and making them feel responsible, at least in part, for any success. In other words, success should be attributed internally.

Top tip

Extended exam questions may ask you to suggest factors that influence a group's potential or to account for faulty processes. Make sure you understand the concept of social loafing and the factors that influence cohesion.

Finally, the coach should set goals for the players and perhaps give them a specific role to play in the game, such as marking a certain opponent or playing in a wider position. Any goals that are set should be realistic and achievable and may represent an improvement on the last performance, such as to make three more tackles.

The Ringlemann effect

This theory suggests that the larger the group the less the collective group effort. Ringlemann performed an experiment using a 'tug of war' trial and discovered that a team of eight did not pull eight times harder than one individual. This suggests that there might be motivational problems in a team when players think that they can leave it to others to cover for them and hide within the team.

Ultimately, cohesion in sport is affected by a constantly changing mix of influences.

Leadership

Some of the most successful teams in sport have won major cups and trophies because they have been managed, coached or captained by an influential leader. Think of the success of Manchester United under the 23-year reign of Sir Alex Ferguson from 1986 until the time of writing.

A leader is someone who can influence others towards achieving goals. There are two types of leader in a sports group:

- An **emergent leader** is one who comes from within the group and assumes responsibility for the role or can be elected by the members of the club. In a sixth-form rounders team it could be that the captain is chosen by the players and coach. He/she is usually a player from year 13 who has played for the team in year 12 and already knows how the team works best. Although unity and the status quo is maintained, there might be a lack of fresh ideas.
- A **prescribed leader** is appointed from outside the group, in the way that the English Football Association appointed Fabio Capello as England manager in 2007. Such a leader may bring a fresh approach and give new impetus to the team, but could disrupt team unity and cause a few upsets. Sometimes players leave a club when a new prescribed leader is appointed.

Key terms

Emergent leader: a leader appointed from within the group.

Prescribed leader: a leader appointed from outside the group.

Leader characteristics: the qualities that facilitate good leadership.

Leaders will emerge or be appointed because they have **leader characteristics**. A good leader will have motivational skills to encourage the team to keep playing when they are losing or are involved in a difficult game. A leader usually has charisma and is well respected by the team. Sometimes the leader needs the ability to empathise — to listen to the needs of the group and to operate with the consensus of opinion. A leader must have good communication skills, so that tactics and strategies are adhered to by all the players. Usually leaders are experienced in their chosen sport and can pass this experience on to others. Finally, a leader should be able to adjust his/her style of leadership to suit the task in hand. There are a number of styles to choose from.

Leadership styles

The **autocratic** or task-oriented style of leadership is when the leader takes charge and dictates to the rest of the group, who have no say in the way the task is undertaken. By contrast, in the **democratic** or person-oriented style of leadership, the leader empathises and listens to the group members before making a decision on how the task should be done.

Key terms

Autocratic style: the leader makes all the decisions and gives the group formal instruction.

Democratic style: the leader listens to the group members and involves them in decision making.

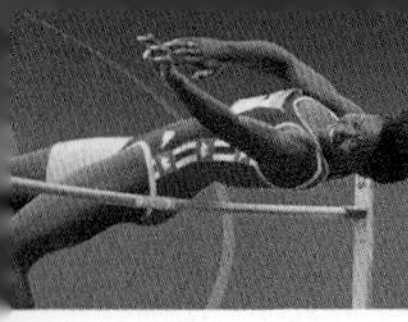

Fiedler's contingency model is summarised in Figure 10.2. According to this model, the choice of either the autocratic or the democratic style depends on how good or how favourable the situation is, and the leader should therefore choose the correct approach according to the situation.

The autocratic style is best when the situation is highly favourable and also when the situation is highly unfavourable. In a favourable situation, the leader is strong and well respected, the task is clear and the team members get on well and understand each other's play. There is no need to spend time discussing tactics, the team accepts and gets on with the decision of the captain. For example, if a netball team has a set play for moving the ball up towards the opposition goal and all the players know this well-rehearsed play, individuals will simply obey the captain's call to execute this move.

An unfavourable situation is one in which the team cannot agree on the tactics to be used, does not follow the instructions from a weak leader, or the task is unclear. A team facing unknown opponents in a hostile away game needs a strong leader to tell them what to do. A group in which the players are uncertain or arguing among themselves may need to be told the best strategy to adopt.

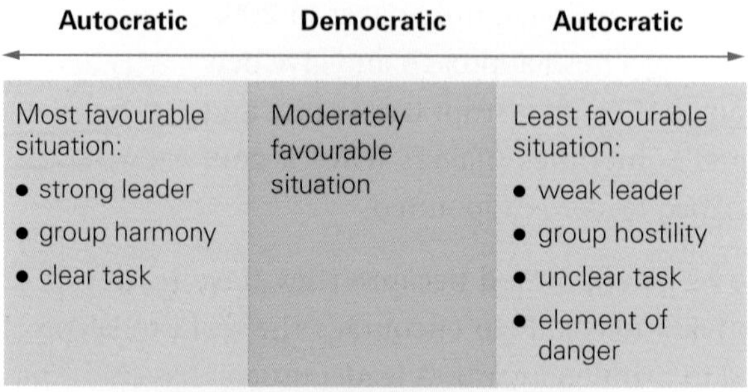

Autocratic	Democratic	Autocratic
Most favourable situation: • strong leader • group harmony • clear task	Moderately favourable situation	Least favourable situation: • weak leader • group hostility • unclear task • element of danger

Figure 10.2 Fiedler's contingency model

The democratic approach is best in a moderate situation, where a group is well established but there is scope for new ideas. In this case it may be best to sit down and discuss tactics with the team before a match.

> **Top tip**
>
> Many exam questions on team dynamics are based on diagrams. Make sure you know and understand the diagrammatic models based on the work of Fiedler and Chelladurai and that you can explain the key phases of each model.

Other styles that the leader can use include the **rewarding style**, when the leader gives incentives such as a player of the match award to motivate the team. Praise and encouragement may also be used to keep the team playing to the best of its ability. A **social support style** involves the coach or captain offering individual advice or feedback to particular players to help them improve their game.

During training sessions, a coach may put the players through their paces by setting up and organising a number of specific skills and drills. This structured and often essential part of leadership is called a **training and instruction style** of leadership.

Sometimes the leader may find it appropriate to take a step back and just let the group get on with it. This laid-back approach is called a **laissez faire style** of leadership. It can be used when the team members are experts in the task and know exactly what they are doing, or when a new coach has been appointed to lead a team and needs to stand back and assess what level his/her new charges are at.

One of the essential qualities of leaders is that they can adapt their leadership style to suit the situation. We have already seen how leaders might choose either the autocratic or the democratic style according to how favourable the situation is, but they may also need to take into account the features of the group or individual they are coaching as well as their own characteristics and preferences before choosing the style in which they want to operate. For example, in a dangerous situation, such as when coaching a contact skill such as a tackle, the leader may want to use an instructive and autocratic style to ensure correct technique and reduce the risk of injury. With beginners, to make sure they learn the basics, the style may be instructive and autocratic, motivational and rewarding. With experts, the leader may step back a little and ask for the democratic input of the group or even let them get on with things in a laissez faire style.

It has therefore been suggested that the best leadership style to use depends on three main influences:

- the situation
- the leader
- the group

Chelladurai's multi-dimensional model (summarised in Figure 10.3) suggests that if the leader can adapt the style of leadership to best fit all three of these influences then it is more likely that a rewarding and satisfactory performance will result. In other words, if the style of leadership chosen is equal to the requirements of the group and the demands of the situation, the better the performance is likely to be.

A final consideration of leadership in sport is the debate over whether leaders are born or made. This debate reflects a nature versus nurture approach to sports psychology. Some argue that people are born with characteristics, such as charisma and motivational skills, that make them

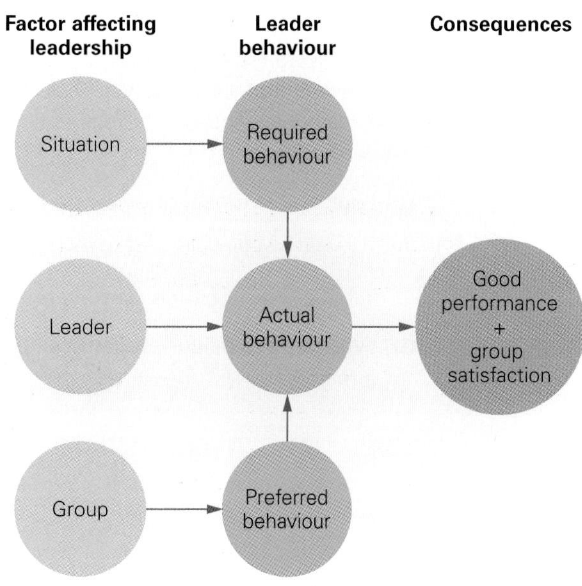

Figure 10.3 Chelladurai's multi-dimensional model of leadership styles

almost natural choices as captains or coaches. Others argue that such characteristics are learned and that good leaders are usually those with experience of the game. Perhaps the best approach is to accept a combination of both nature and nurture theories — that leaders are indeed born with essential leadership characteristics and that these characteristics are used in accordance with the circumstances under which the group will operate.

Tasks to tackle 10.3

Look again at the styles of leadership listed on pages 85–87. For each style, give a sporting situation in which you would use that style, and give a reason for your choice. For example, you might choose to use an autocratic style of leadership in a dangerous situation, such as swimming, especially if you were coaching beginners.

Top tip

It is essential that you know the situations in which autocratic and democratic leadership styles are used and that you can describe what you mean by a favourable and an unfavourable situation. Make sure that when you answer a question on the factors influencing leadership style you include not only situational factors but also the influence of the group and the leader's characteristics. Make sure that you give an example and an explanation from each of the three influences on leadership according to Chelladurai, namely situation, leader and group.

Practice makes perfect

1 Elite performers sometimes train on their own and sometimes as part of a group. How would you distinguish between a group and a collection of individuals? *(3 marks)*

2 Team players are often influenced by a leader who helps them to achieve an active and healthy lifestyle. Distinguish between a prescribed and an emergent leader and describe the characteristics that may be necessary for effective leadership in sport. *(5 marks)*

3 (a) Look at this model of group performance:

actual productivity = potential productivity – faulty processes

What is meant by the term potential productivity? *(1 mark)*

(b) What are the influences that can combine to produce faulty processes in a team? *(3 marks)*

Chapter 11 Emotional control of sporting performance

Psychological aspects that optimise performance

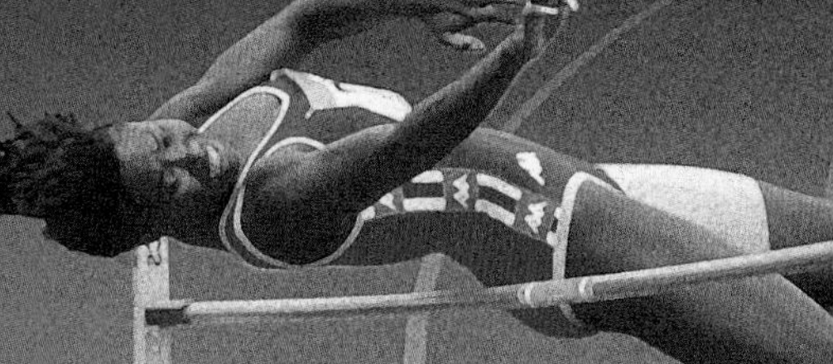

What you need to know

By the end of this chapter you should be able to:

- say how confidence can affect sporting performance
- describe why and how coaches set goals for their performers
- understand the importance of controlling emotions such as anxiety and stress in sport

Confidence in sport

Confidence can be defined as a belief in your ability to master a particular situation. There are three factors that affect the level of confidence shown by a sports performer: personality, experience and situation. For example, a professional footballer playing in a European cup competition may be worried if his team is due to play the away leg of the cup tie at a ground at which he has never played before. The situation may be new to him; however, his experience of playing in many European competitions may help to reduce such lack of confidence, especially if the player is **competitive** and has a naturally confident personality. In other words, these three major influences on confidence can combine to produce a level of confidence in any given sporting situation.

> **Key terms**
>
> **Competitiveness:** the degree to which challenging situations are welcomed.
>
> **Trait confidence:** an innate degree of self-belief in being able to master a situation.
>
> **State confidence:** a temporary degree of self-belief in a given situation.

Confidence can be an innate personality characteristic. This is **trait confidence**, which is general and consistent. **State confidence** can change depending on the situation and the performer's past success in that situation.

Self-efficacy theory

While confidence refers to a general predisposition, confidence in any given sporting situation can be referred to as **self-efficacy**. The psychologist Bandura suggested that self-efficacy depends on four factors:

- **Performance accomplishments** — this refers to the amount of success that performers have achieved in the past on a similar task. For example, at an athletics meeting, a high jumper who has cleared 1.25 m in a recent training session will be confident of clearing the bar that is currently set at 1.10 m.

- **Vicarious experience** — this relates to players seeing others, especially their peers, perform a task similar to the one they are about to do themselves. Essentially, if someone else can do it, so can you! For example, at a junior school swimming lesson, the children may be apprehensive of diving in at the deep end despite the expert instruction of the teacher who is building the dive up from a sitting position. However, when one of the class attempts the dive successfully, the rest may be less apprehensive about having a go.
- **Verbal persuasion** — this relates to the amount of encouragement received from significant others, such as a coach, friends or family members. For example, you might feel a lot calmer when approaching a major event if your coach comments on how well you have been doing in training and that he/she knows you can perform well on the day of the event.
- **Emotional arousal** — this refers to the level of anxiety that a player may experience leading up to a big game. Ways of controlling such high levels of anxiety are discussed later in this chapter.

Bandura argued that if the four self-efficacy factors are positive, the performer will believe that he/she can do well and will succeed.

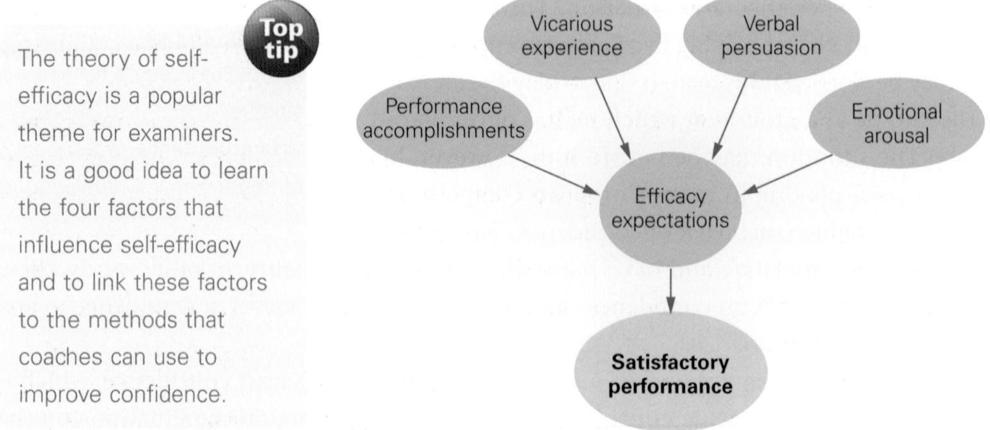

Top tip
The theory of self-efficacy is a popular theme for examiners. It is a good idea to learn the four factors that influence self-efficacy and to link these factors to the methods that coaches can use to improve confidence.
Vicarious experience
Verbal persuasion
Performance accomplishments
Emotional arousal
Efficacy expectations
Satisfactory performance

Figure 11.1 Bandura's self-efficacy theory

Improving self-efficacy

A lack of confidence can lead to anxiety and nervousness in sport, and performance can be adversely affected if confidence is low. Coaches should therefore understand the many influences that affect confidence in sport and should be careful to use a range of strategies to promote confidence in their players.

To promote confidence relating to performance accomplishments, the coach can highlight past successes of the player(s) and the performance failures of the opposition. For example,

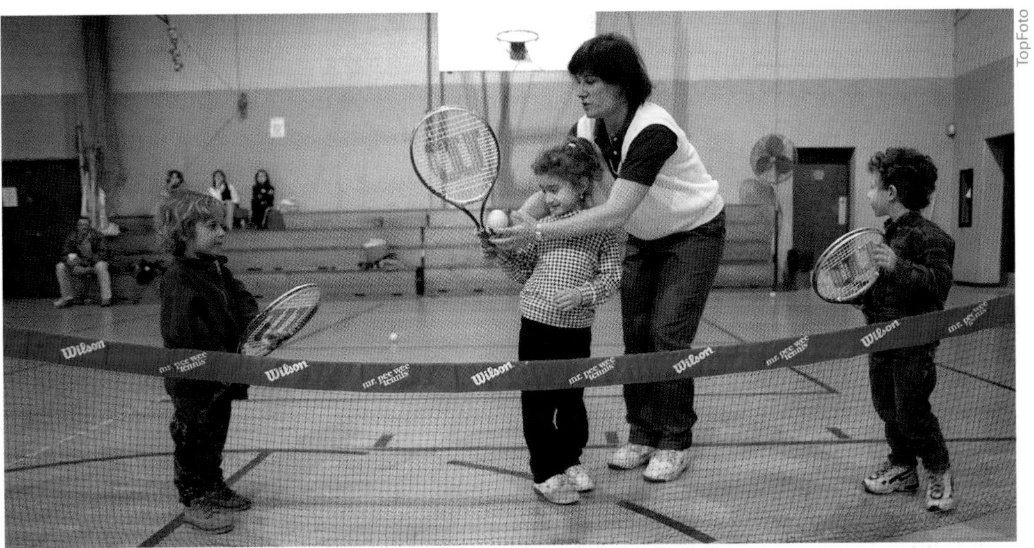

TopFoto

'Junior' versions of sports ensure successful performance accomplishments

the coach of a football team about to play the second round of a cup may point out that the opposing team has already been beaten in the league this season. When coaching beginners, the coach should make sure that success is achieved at an early stage by setting tasks that are within the capabilities of the players. For example, when coaching passing skills in team games, the coach might ask for the pass to be practised without any opposition in a static situation before introducing the pressure of an opponent in the passing drill.

An accurate demonstration of the skills and tactics to be used in the game can increase confidence relating to vicarious experience. The coach may also point out other players who are successfully performing similar tasks and these players can be used as **role models**. The coach should be careful to use role models to which the players in their charge can aspire. If top-class professionals are used as role models for beginners, the beginners might think that they could never be that good and actually lose confidence.

Positive verbal persuasion can be used by the coach in the lead-up to a game. Offering encouragement and praise, and telling performers that others think they will succeed can often help to improve confidence. The coach can also offer encouragement through rewards and incentives, such as player of the match awards. A final way to promote confidence is to make it clear to the players that any success achieved is down to them rather than due to any external influences. Success at an athletics meeting could be attributed to the effort put in by the athlete rather than the below-par performance of his/her competitors.

Key term

Role models: people we regard in high esteem who set targets and abilities we would aspire to match.

Tasks to tackle 11.1

List the four considerations that make up self-efficacy theory. For each factor that you list, suggest a method that the coach could use to develop and promote its influence.

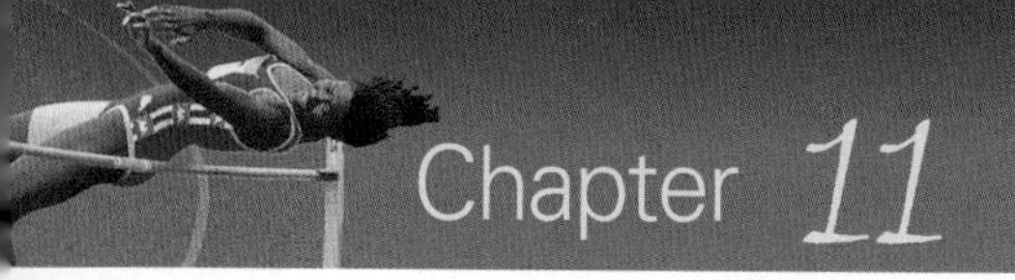

To promote confidence, the coach should lower the anxiety and emotional arousal felt by performers. A good way to do this is to practise mentally before the competition (see p. 97–98), allowing the players to go through the performance in their mind several times before the big day. A gymnast might mentally run through the sequence of the routine before performing in a competition to make sure that the order of skills is correct. Emotional arousal and anxiety can also be controlled by muscular relaxation techniques (see p. 99).

Goal setting in sport

Various research studies into sports psychology have found a positive link between goal setting and improved performance. Players who set themselves achievable targets or who have goals set by their coach generally produce better results. The specific boundaries established by such targets give players something to aim for, so that personal motivation is provided and a sense of satisfaction is felt when that target is achieved. Confidence will improve once a goal has been reached, allowing a more difficult target to be set to allow further improvement. Goal setting also has an important role in lowering anxiety and reducing the stress of performing at a high level.

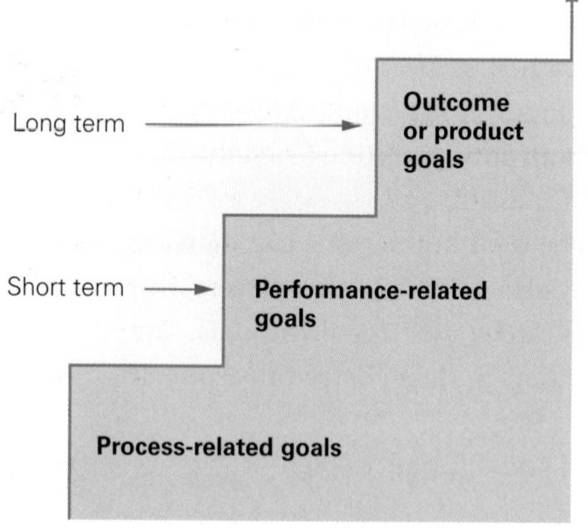

Figure 11.2 A summary of the types of goal that can be set by players and coaches

The goals set by coaches and players can be long term or short term. Long-term goals are concerned with the end result of a lengthy period of work and are sometimes called **outcome goals**. For example, an outcome goal for a swimmer may be to qualify for regional team selection. Short-term goals are the stepping-stones towards meeting long-term targets. **Performance goals** are short term and are judged against a past performance. For example, an attempt by a swimmer to beat her personal best time by the end of next month might be a step towards meeting the regional target time. **Process goals** are concerned with technique and are also short term. For example, in order to achieve a personal best, the swimmer must work on improving her exit from each turn.

It is important that goals do not focus solely on winning. In an athletics race, for example, there can only be one winner and performers who fail to meet that target may lose motivation and suffer stress. It is more important to set goals that can be achieved, such as those that focus on personal improvement and technique. Personal goals provide intrinsic motivation and a sense of satisfaction from doing your best.

Key terms

Outcome goals: the end result after a lengthy period of work.

Performance goals: targets related to improvement and enhancing current standards.

Process goals: targets related to improving technique.

An athlete may not win the race but can still gain a personal best time and show improved technique.

Other factors that a coach might consider when setting goals are summed up by the **SMARTER** principle. This is a set of guidelines that should be taken into account when setting goals. Goals should be:

Specific — 'going up one level on the bleep test' is a specific goal, 'improving fitness' is not.

Measured — statistics or a stopwatch should be used to inform performers about their achievement.

Agreed —players should sit down and discuss the goals with the coach, so that they are involved in the goal-setting process.

Realistic — the goals should offer a challenge but be achievable.

Timed — a goal should be long term or short term, and preferably have a specific date, in order to help keep the performer focused.

Exciting — players work harder for something they are interested in.

Recorded — progress should be written down to allow for evaluation.

If the SMARTER principle is followed, then improved performance and confidence should follow.

Tasks to tackle 11.2

Goal setting is an important technique that coaches and players can use to improve their performance. In your own sport, think of a long-term objective or outcome goal that you would like to achieve this season and then suggest some shorter-term goals that would help you to achieve your aim.

Top tip

Maximising the effectiveness of goal setting is a popular topic with examiners. Do learn the SMARTER principle, but don't forget that effective goal setting does not always mean setting a target to win — performance and process goals are also important.

Anxiety and stress in sport

One of the most common reasons for failure in sports performance is high stress and anxiety levels in the athlete. In simple terms, when you are nervous your performance is not as good. In sports psychology it is important to look at the causes of stress and anxiety to see if anything can be done to prevent or reduce the symptoms of stress.

The terms stress and anxiety are linked. **Stress** can be defined as the response of the body to a threatening situation. The causes of stress, known as stressors, may be perceived by the performer either positively or negatively, and it is the performer's **perception** that dictates the response to the threat. For example, at the start of a race, an athlete becomes aware that some of the runners have faster personal best times than he does. The response to this competitive threat could be positive: 'I've been training well and I think I can use the faster

Key terms

Stress: the response (not always negative) of the body to a threat.

Perception: what we think might happen; not necessarily what does happen.

Anxiety: the negative response to a threat, including irrational thinking and worry.

Concentration: the ability to maintain attention on the required task.

Top tip

Learn the difference between anxiety, stress and arousal because these basic definitions are often required in the exam and they can gain you a couple of easy marks.

pace to up my own personal best.' However, the response to this threat could be negative: 'These runners have got really fast times and I've got no chance of winning today!'

Such positive or negative responses determine the confidence and motivation levels of the athlete. A positive response to a stressor could actually improve motivation and result in an enhanced performance, so stress should not always be viewed negatively — it can help to produce better results. When the response to a stressor is negative, it becomes anxiety. **Anxiety** is the negative aspect of stress characterised by irrational thinking, worry and loss of **concentration**.

In sport, stress — and by consequence anxiety if the stressor is perceived in a negative way — can be caused by a number of influences. Highly competitive situations can be stressors, such as playing in a cup final or a major event such as a regional championship. Performers may be aware that higher levels of effort and technique are needed in order to succeed. Are they up to the task? Stress and anxiety can also be caused by the anticipation of conflict in sport. For example, the possibility of being marked by a strong and robust player who is known to play to the limit of the rules may cause apprehension before the game starts. Frustration is another stressor, often caused by the same factors that lead to aggression in sport, perhaps by being fouled, not playing well or losing. Such frustration causes the blood pressure and heart rate to go up. Another cause of stress is climatic influences. Playing a fast, physical sport in very hot conditions increases heart rates and levels of fatigue. Rugby league, for example, is played in the summer months when temperatures can reach over 40°C.

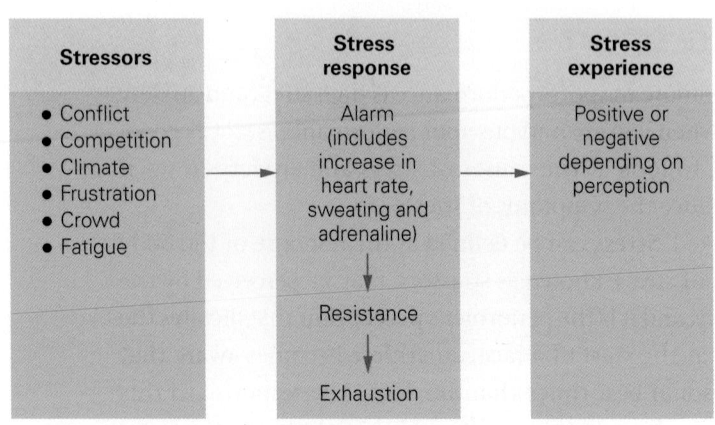

Figure 11.3 Features of stress in sport

Remember that in all these stressful situations it is the players' perception of how they can meet the demands of the situation that is important. If they think they can match the threat, then a good performance should result; if they feel they are unable to match the threat, then anxiety and an inhibited performance may occur. Figure 11.3 shows that the stressors discussed above can cause an athlete some initial shock or alarm but then it is the athlete who determines whether to treat the stressor in a positive or negative way.

Anxiety

Anxiety is an unwelcome feature of sports performance. Performers may view a situation negatively and begin to think irrationally. Worrying thoughts may enter their mind, such as 'What if I get injured today playing against this overly physical team?' or 'If I miss this penalty I will let everyone down'. They might worry about events well before the game takes place, such as not meeting the demands of the training schedule, or even about matters unconnected with sport, such as family concerns. The effect of all this is that they begin to lose concentration on the task and become tense and lacking in confidence.

Anxiety may be experienced in two ways. Anxiety that occurs in the mind, or psychological anxiety, is known as **cognitive anxiety**. Physiological anxiety is known as **somatic anxiety**. Somatic anxiety is characterised by the physical responses of the body to stressors such as an increase in heart rate, a rise in adrenaline levels, increased sweating, muscular tension and poor coordination.

The relationship between these two types of anxiety is important, and is depicted by two graphs as shown in Figures 11.4 and 11.5.

Figure 11.4 shows that somatic anxiety can have a positive effect on performance initially. The increased adrenaline and awareness may produce more effort. However, further increases in somatic anxiety will cause performance to deteriorate. The effects of cognitive anxiety are much more detrimental to the player. As the graph shows, the more you worry, the worse you play. The best performance tends to occur when cognitive anxiety is at its lowest.

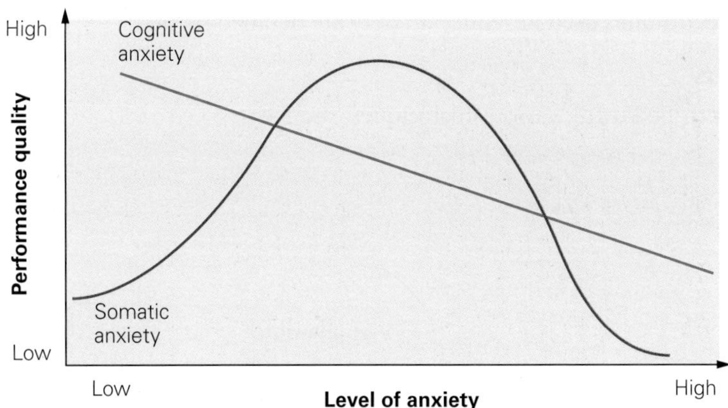

Figure 11.4 The relationship between cognitive anxiety, somatic anxiety and performance

Key terms

Cognitive anxiety: psychological anxiety, worry in the mind.

Somatic anxiety: physiological anxiety, physical symptoms of stress.

Top tip

The graph shown in Figure 11.4 sometimes appears in exams. Learn the different levels of cognitive and somatic anxiety that can occur in the lead-up to an event and use the graph to remind you of your knowledge.

Note that the shape of the somatic anxiety curve in this graph is almost identical to the one that shows the relationship between arousal and performance, called the 'inverted U', which is discussed later in this chapter.

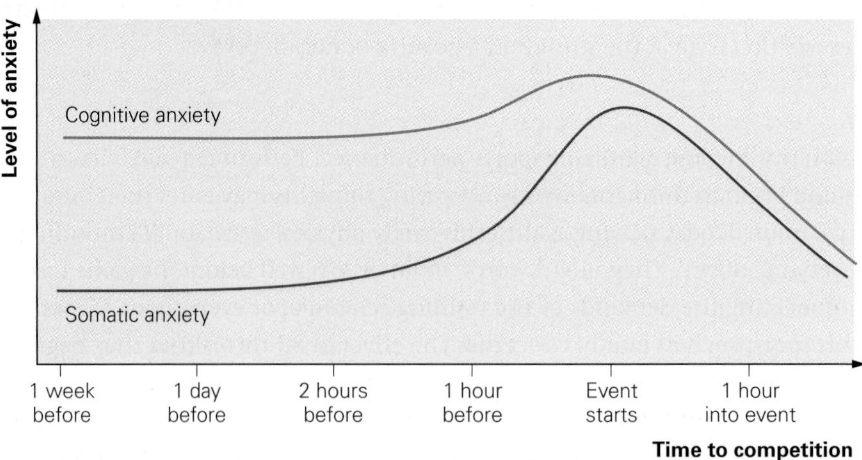

Figure 11.5 The relationship between anxiety and the time approaching competition

Figure 11.5 also shows differences between cognitive and somatic anxiety but this time the differences are concerned with the timing of the mental and physical responses to anxiety. Somatic anxiety tends to surface in the hours leading up to a major competition and peaks just before the event takes place. Once the competition is underway, somatic anxiety tends to decline. Cognitive anxiety tends to be high well before the event and again peaks just before play starts. Cognitive anxiety then fluctuates once the match is underway in response to success or failure.

The implications for the coach of the differences between cognitive and somatic anxiety in the days prior to competition are very significant. Cognitive anxieties may be present well before the event is due to take place. Since the feelings associated with cognitive anxiety are internal, the coach may be unaware that the player is suffering from them. All sports coaches should try to reduce the effects of anxiety, and in particular cognitive anxiety, well before major sporting events. The techniques used to reduce anxiety are detailed below.

Reducing cognitive anxiety

Cognitive anxiety can be controlled using various techniques, such as:

- visualisation
- imagery
- mental rehearsal
- positive self-talk
- thought stopping
- goal setting

> Key term
>
> **Visualisation:** creating a mental picture of a successful attempt to complete a task as if in a real situation.

Visualisation involves picturing yourself doing the skill that you are practising in a competitive situation. For example, a football player might be taking free kicks successfully in practice, but when it comes to the actual game on a Saturday afternoon those free kicks are not as good. What the player needs to do is to imagine during the training session that the free kicks are being taken for real, perhaps when there is more pressure, more fatigue and in the presence of a crowd. The player needs to feel any anticipated sources of anxiety and overcome them so that when it comes to actually taking the free kicks for real, any stressors have been dealt with in practice. A successful attempt in training should be locked into the thoughts of the player so that it can be repeated for real. Having dealt with the anxiety already, the player should maintain confidence and produce better end results.

Top tip

Visualisation, imagery and mental rehearsal are similar, so make sure you know the how to differentiate between them.

Another method of controlling cognitive anxiety is **imagery**. This is similar to visualisation in that the performer pictures in his mind a successful attempt at the skill. This time, however, the performer looks back at an earlier task or game, one in which he/she performed well — perhaps a cup-winning performance or a game that led to the award of player of the match. The key is to try to recreate the sense of pride gained from a past success so that more confidence and less anxiety is felt at the present time. The idea is to tell yourself 'I did it before, so I can do it again'.

Key terms

Imagery: recreating a mental picture of a task that has been successfully completed in the past.

Mental rehearsal: going over a performance in the mind repeatedly.

Mental rehearsal involves going over a practised skill, drill or routine in the mind without physical movement so that the sequence of actions is stored firmly in the memory. Mental rehearsal is very useful when performing serial skills involving a sequence of well-learned movements, such as those required when performing a gym routine. Such movements are performed in a set order and this set routine can be rehearsed before competition. Closed skills, when the sequence of movements is not likely to change, are well-suited to mental rehearsal since it is unlikely that the performer will have to alter the pre-learned sequence.

Mental rehearsal can be used by both novice and experienced players. In the case of a novice, the coach could use mental rehearsal in small chunks as part of a distributed practice session. For example, when the player is resting the coach could remind him/her of basic techniques to run through in their mind. In the case of an expert, the coach might allow the player time to devote to the whole task or sequence, concentrating on detail and repeating the finer aspects of the task in the mind over and over again.

In all three cognitive management techniques mentioned above there are considerations that both coaches and players should note to make the techniques successful. First, the coach should take into account the level of experience of the player, so that the mental techniques can be applied in a different manner for the novice and the expert, as explained above. When any of the cognitive techniques are used they should always concentrate on success. The player should visualise performing the task with a successful end result or imagine a previous winning performance. Players should use real time when using mental rehearsal. Real time refers to the actual time it takes to perform the task in competition, so that if a gym routine lasts for 85 seconds then that is the time the gymnast must spend mentally rehearsing the routine. When a player is mentally rehearsing, visualising or using imagery, it is a good idea to avoid distractions, so a quiet space without any disturbance should be used.

When mental practice is used successfully it can have a positive effect on performance. Studies have measured the performances of athletes who performed an unfamiliar task by (a) mentally practising only, (b) using physical practice only and (c) by doing both physical and mental practice. The best results were achieved by those who did both mental and physical practice. Mental practice reduces anxiety, improves confidence and provides motivation.

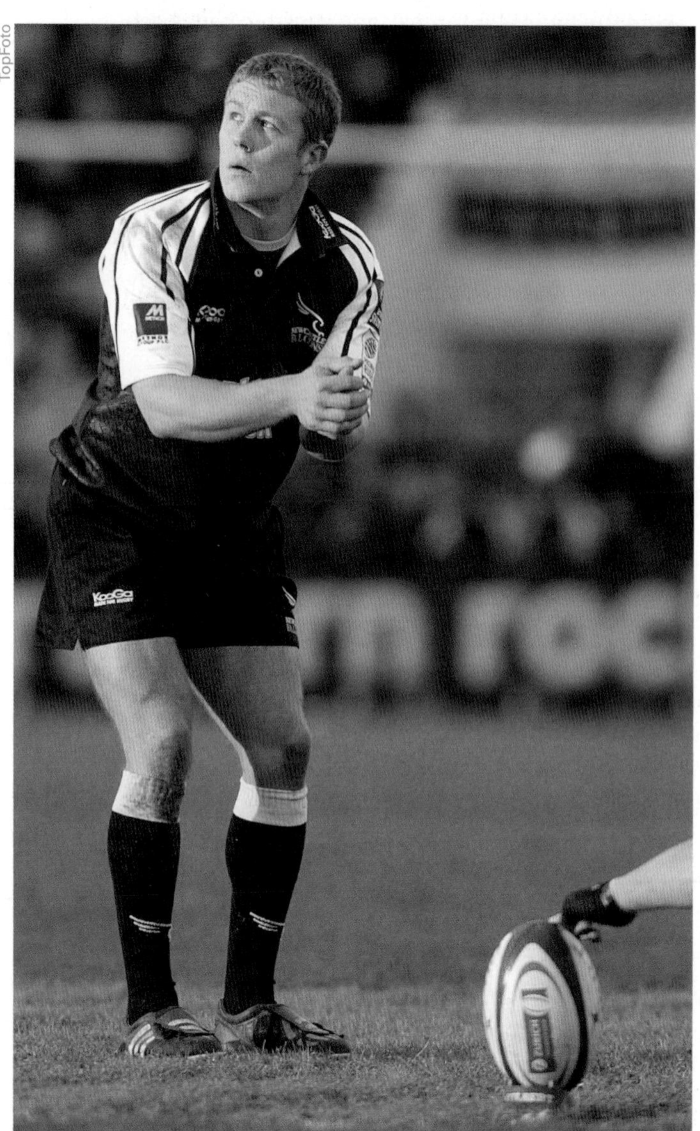

TopFoto

Jonny Wilkinson's trademark visualisation and self-talk before attempting a conversion have been much copied

Other methods of controlling anxiety can be used specifically during performance. **Positive self-talk** involves athletes reminding themselves what they need to do to succeed. When you watch a rugby union kicker line up an attempt at goal, you will probably see him take a deep breath and you may notice his lips move just before he takes the kick. The player is using positive self-talk to remind himself of the technique needed to make a successful attempt. Positive self-talk can be used to remind a player of tactics and strategies given by the coach before the game; it can be used to break bad habits so that the performer does not

Key term

Positive self-talk: reminding yourself of important information or replacing negative thoughts with positive ones.

keep repeating a poor play; or it can be used to concentrate on weaknesses in the opponent or a strength in the performer's own play. 'Stop that daft shot' or 'Concentrate on the back-hand' are comments that players may make to themselves.

Thought stopping is another technique used by players to prevent negative thinking from hindering performance. Thoughts such as 'I can't do that shot' are deliberately put to one side.

Goal setting, as we have already seen, can also be used to control anxiety because it allows players to meet targets and gain confidence when a target is met. Improved confidence is usually a measure of lower anxiety.

Reducing somatic anxiety

Somatic anxiety is physical, so the coach or player can use the following techniques:

Progressive relaxation techniques can be used to relieve muscular tension. The athlete is guided through a series of static tensing exercises that involve holding a particular group of muscles at maximum contraction for a short period of time and then gradually releasing the hold. Each part of the body is worked on in turn, starting with the periphery and working towards the body core. The athlete can learn to concentrate on tension reduction, and once the technique is learned, the tension caused by anxiety can be dramatically reduced.

Breathing techniques can also be used to counter physical anxiety. Here the athlete attempts a series of controlled breathing exercises to help them slow their breathing rate and focus on the task. You will often see a football player take a deep breath before attempting a penalty kick.

Biofeedback uses physical measurements to record the reduction in anxiety that can be achieved by the methods mentioned above. For example, a heart monitor could be used to measure the reduction in heart rate achieved by using imagery, visualisation or self-talk. When the results of the different methods are compared, the athlete will know which method works best for them. Biofeedback is therefore a physical way of testing which anxiety counter method — be it somatic or cognitive — is best for them.

Other types of anxiety

Some sports performers tend to worry most of the time, even if there is only a small chance of the things they are concerned about actually happening. Such naturally anxious athletes are said to show **trait anxiety**. Trait anxiety is inherent, consistent and enduring. The athlete will continue to worry in most situations and the coach should use the anxiety control methods outlined above to help reduce both cognitive and somatic anxieties.

State anxiety is more temporary but equally significant. It occurs in specific situations, such as taking a penalty, or serving for the match in tennis, when a

> **Key terms**
>
> **Trait anxiety:** an innate characteristic of inherent worry and lack of self-belief.
>
> **State anxiety:** a temporary lack of self-belief in a given situation.

rush of anxious thoughts and physical tension, or loss of concentration, may result in a poor performance. You may have witnessed missed penalties in shoot outs or tennis players who fail to close out the match at match point.

The effects of anxiety are amplified if naturally anxious performers are placed in situations that may cause more anxiety. In other words, players who have the trait are more likely to show state anxiety. The combination of trait and state anxiety can lead to well below par performance. The manager or coach should find out which players are likely to find specific situations stressful by testing them for anxiety before major competitions, so that such players can avoid the threat.

Top tip

The terms 'trait' and 'state' appear more then once in this section of the course, so make sure that you know what these terms mean so that you can use them correctly.

Tasks to tackle 11.3

Make a list of some of the influences that you think could cause anxiety and stress in sport and give an example for each influence that you list.

Measuring anxiety

A number of anxiety tests have been developed that are specifically targeted at sports competition. The **sport competition anxiety test**, or SCAT test, designed by the psychologist Martens, is the best known of these, but you may also see the names SCA1 and CSAI2.

The SCAT test is a questionnaire in which athletes are asked to answer a series of questions by ticking a box and are then given a rating as to their level of anxiety in sporting competition. The test, an example of which is given below, has the same advantages and disadvantages as other personality tests discussed in Chapter 9. In an attempt to avoid the problem of biased answers, some of the questions are unrelated to the subject matter so that the real subject being tested — anxiety — is masked. Have a go at the test and see how you rate. The method of calculating your score is shown at the end of the test.

Statements	Hardly ever	Sometimes	Often
(1) Competing against others is socially enjoyable			
(2) Before I compete I feel uneasy			
(3) Before I compete I worry about not playing well			
(4) I am a good sportsperson when I compete			
(5) When I compete I worry about making mistakes			
(6) Before I compete I am calm			
(7) Setting a goal is important when competing			
(8) Before I compete I get a queasy feeling in my stomach			
(9) Just before competing I notice my heart beats faster than usual			

How to score the test:

- Items 1, 4 and 7 do not count (they are designed to mask the test).
- Score items 2, 3, 5, 8 and 9 as: hardly ever = 1, sometimes = 2, often = 3
- Score item 6 as: hardly ever = 3, sometimes = 2, often = 1

The maximum score is 18. The higher the score, the higher is the competitive anxiety. Is this a quick and easy method of assessing personality?

The relationship between arousal and performance

Arousal is defined as the level of readiness to perform. It prepares the body for action and includes an increase in adrenaline levels, an increase in heart rate and a muscular anticipation. However, too much or too little arousal can have a detrimental effect on performance. Increased arousal can be caused by the approach of a major competition or big game, by others watching the performance (especially if those watching are knowledgeable about the sport, such as a chief scout from a local club, or if they are significant others), by increasingly frustrating circumstances (such as being fouled), or by a fear of failure. When an increase in arousal occurs, the effect on performance is explained by a number of theories.

Key term

Arousal: the degree of activation and readiness to perform a task.

Drive theory

Drive theory suggests that as the level of arousal increases, so performance improves in a linear or constant fashion. It is explained by the following formula:

$$P = D \times H$$

In other words, performance is the product of drive and habit.

It is suggested that an athlete is initially motivated by the challenge of meeting the task or by the big game, and that the increased effort put in brings success, and the drive to continue performing. The success achieved provides reinforcement and the athlete carries on repeating the successful responses so that the performance becomes habitual. Drive theory is depicted in Figure 11.6, which shows performance improving continuously with increasing arousal.

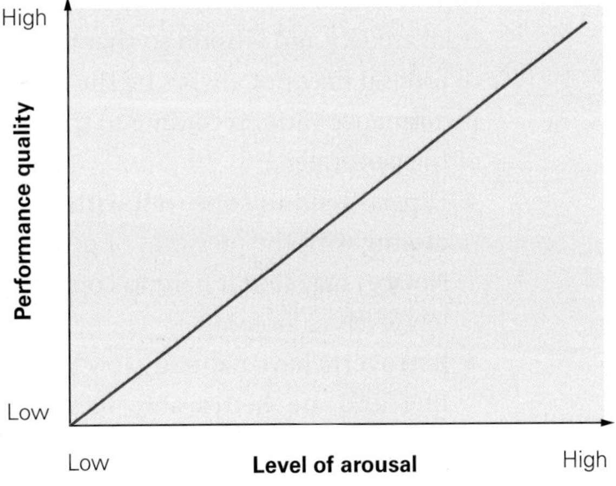

Figure 11.6 Drive theory

Top tip

Exam questions often ask you to describe the relationship between arousal and performance. Make sure that you can sketch the graphs and that you know all the key points that relate to each theory: drive theory, inverted U theory, drive reduction and catastrophe theory. Extra marks can often be gained by giving an explanation of the dominant response and how it affects drive theory and for suggesting that a moderate level of arousal may not always be the most beneficial level of arousal.

However, at high levels of arousal the ability to take in information from the environment is reduced and performers may only focus on the **dominant response**, or the most intense stimulus. Expert performers may be able to continue playing well at high arousal because they can focus on the correct dominant response using their experience, but novices may focus on an incorrect response and their performance could suffer.

Drive reduction theory

This theory suggests that motivation is high at the start of the learning process, when performers are challenged by the need to master the task, but that once success has been achieved that initial drive is lost — the need has been satisfied. The drive to master the task and overcome the challenge is replaced by a sense of satisfaction based on successful completion of the skill. A new challenge or an extension to the skill is needed to provide further motivation.

The inverted U theory

The inverted U theory states that increases in arousal can improve performance up to an optimum point, which occurs at a moderate level of arousal. Further increases in arousal have a detrimental effect on performance. Therefore, both low and high levels of arousal can produce a performance that is below our best. At low arousal, performers may be under-activated and not sufficiently motivated. At high arousal, performers may begin to suffer from anxiety and tension so that their performance is inhibited. However, a moderate level of arousal may not always be the most productive. The best level of arousal for optimum performance varies according to the task being attempted and the personality and expertise of the performer.

- Experts tend to cope well with high levels of arousal because they are experienced at dealing with the pressures of performance, for example playing in front of a large crowd. Novices may find it hard to cope with the increased pressure and tend to perform best at low levels of arousal.
- **Extroverts** have naturally low levels of adrenaline and are better able to cope with the increases in adrenaline levels associated with arousal than **introverts**, who already have high adrenaline levels.

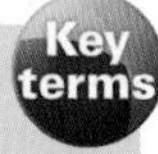

Introvert: a quiet and reserved personality.

Extrovert: a loud and bright personality.

The amount of stimulation required to provoke increases in arousal and adrenaline is determined by the **reticular activating system**. The reticular activating system (RAS) is the part of the brain believed to be the centre of arousal and motivation in mammals. It brings relevant information to our attention and acts like a filter between the conscious and the subconscious.

- Simple tasks require little decision making and can be performed at higher arousal levels than complex tasks. At high levels of arousal, fewer decisions are attempted because fewer items of information are processed in the brain. Decisions at high arousal are based on limited information. A simple task such as a forward roll can therefore be attempted at high arousal. However, at low arousal we may be more able to make the decisions required for complex skills because more information can be processed.
- Gross skills can be performed at high arousal because they require less control and more muscular involvement. Finer skills require more control and are best performed at low arousal levels. For example, a rugby tackle can be attempted with a higher level of arousal than a badminton drop shot.

Key term

RAS: the reticular activating system (RAS) is a function of the brain to release amounts of adrenaline.

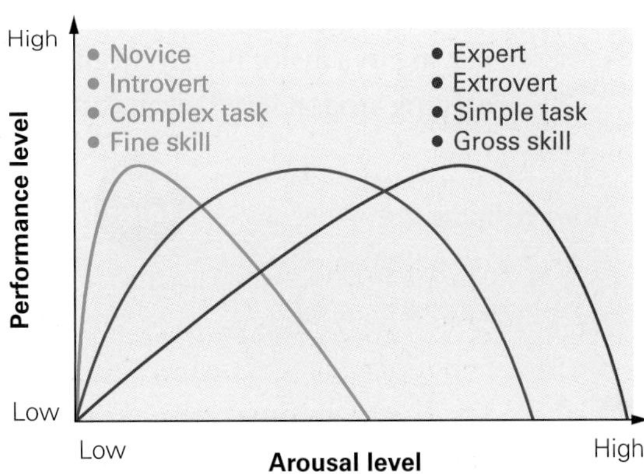

Figure 11.7 The inverted U theory and how it can be adapted to take account of the task and the performer

Top tip

Don't be put off in the exam if you see a graph. The answers to the question can be contained in it!

Cue utilisation hypothesis

Key term

Cue utilisation: the degree to which the performer can use information from the environment.

Easterbrook suggests that the number of environmental cues we can process is related to our level of arousal. In an adaptation of the inverted U theory, he suggests that at low levels of arousal the performer has the capacity to take in a relatively large amount of information but that this wide range of cues may cause confusion and result in a lower level of performance. At high arousal performance may also be at a lower level because the performer tends to concentrate on less information and therefore important cues may be missed. At moderate arousal, however, performance tends to be at a high level because the player concentrates on just the right amount of information and picks up all the relevant cues. Since this theory suggests that a moderate level of arousal produces the best performance, it supports the ideas outlined in the inverted U theory.

Catastrophe theory

This adapted version of the inverted U theory explains why even the best attempts to control arousal levels can suddenly be undermined in sport. Increases in arousal improve performance up to a certain point but then, rather than a gradual decline in performance, a further increase in arousal pushes the performer over the edge and performance falls dramatically. It may only take a small increase in arousal to reach this point of **catastrophe** but this small increase, caused perhaps by a worry about not playing well, by the threat of a difficult opponent or by playing in a major final in front of a big crowd, can have a cumulative effect. When added to existing arousal levels, even experts can experience this kind of disaster.

Key term

Catastrophe: a dramatic and severe deterioration in performance.

Changes in the situation can cause a sufficient increase in arousal to invoke a catastrophe. Imagine a tennis player who wins the semi-final of a major tournament. She has been playing her best tennis and knows she has a chance of winning in the final. On the day of the final, she plays great tennis in the first set, taking it to a tie-break. She then begins to feel the pressure of the moment and suddenly her performance plummets.

The catastrophe is caused by a combination of cognitive and somatic anxieties — the internal worries about not playing well are compounded by physical effects such as muscular tension. To get over the catastrophe the performer must return to a level of arousal that was present before the catastrophe occurred — a feat not always possible under extreme pressure.

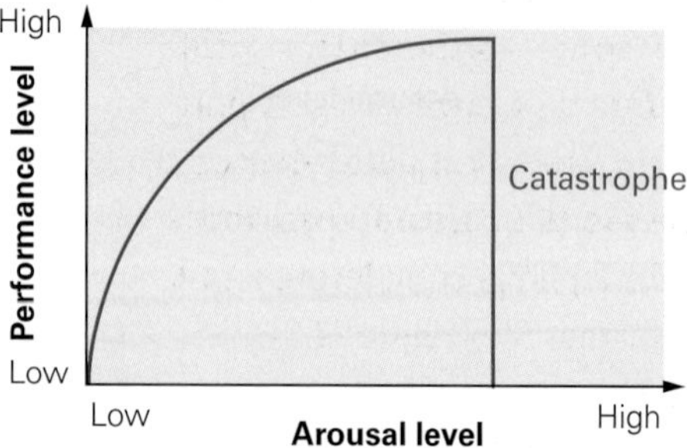

Figure 11.8 Catastrophe theory

The zone

Sometimes, athletes reach a level of performance that is both anxiety free and technically near perfect. They reach what is known as the **zone**, or zone of optimal functioning. The zone is characterised by feelings of calm despite the intense pressure. A sense of supreme confidence exists and the performer is almost totally immersed in the action, with concentration levels at an all-time high. The resultant performance is near perfect, with few errors, lots of energy and correct decision making — the whole event seems to flow in a smooth, efficient manner.

Key term

The zone: an energised, yet controlled, frame of mind that is focused on the task.

The zone is obviously a state the performer will want to achieve. It is usually associated with top-level athletes who have perfected and practised the anxiety control measures of visualisation, imagery, self-talk and mental rehearsal discussed earlier in this chapter.

The zone of optimal functioning (ZOF), proposed by the psychologist Hanin, is another adaptation of the inverted

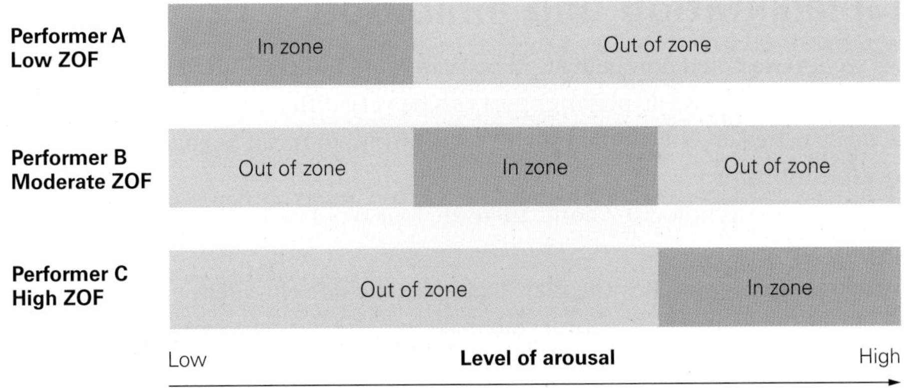

Figure 11.9 Summary showing how the zone of optimal functioning varies for individual performers

U theory. Like the inverted U theory, it suggests that the optimum level of arousal varies depending on the type of task being performed and the person performing it. However, the best level of arousal for each situation is depicted by an area — or zone — rather than a point.

The theory suggests that a novice or a person performing a fine task, such as a golf putt, operates best at a low arousal zone (performer A in Figure 11.9). An expert performer or a player performing a gross skill, such as a tackle, requires a higher level of arousal (performer C in Figure 11.9). A moderate level of arousal may be suitable for a player completing a task that requires a degree of control, such as a volleyball block (performer B in Figure 11.9).

The best performance can be achieved when the challenge of the task is appropriate to the performer's skill. According to Figure 11.10, which shows the **peak flow experience**, players who have little skill and are presented with a difficult task will suffer anxiety. For example, novice rock climbers would be nervous if they were asked to ascend a difficult route. Players with little skill who are offered no challenge will be apathetic to the task. Skilled players who are asked to do an easy task that is well below their capability will quickly become bored. For example, a young experienced swimmer who trains five mornings a week would not relish the basic demands of a school swimming lesson for beginners. To produce a top performance and achieve peak flow, skilled players should be set a task that is difficult enough to challenge them and offers a real incentive for success.

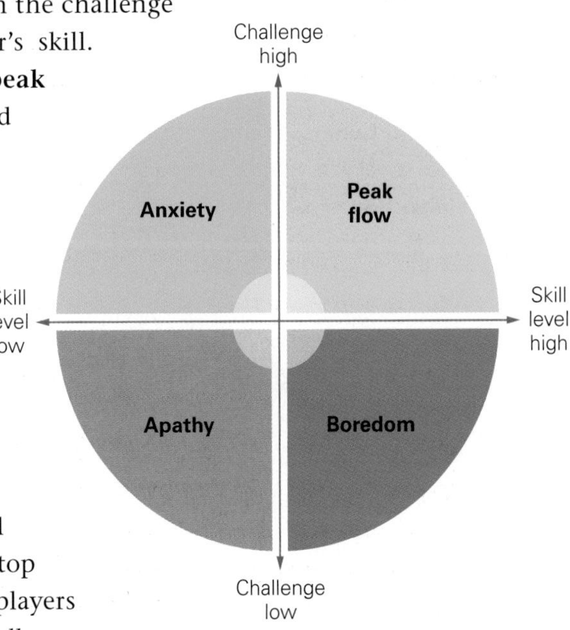

Figure 11.10 Peak flow experience

Social facilitation and inhibition

In the last section we noted how being watched can cause a distraction to the performer. The effects of being watched while playing sport can be very different — the performance can either be made better, an effect called **social facilitation**, or it can be made worse, an effect called **social inhibition**.

According to the psychologist Zajonc, there are four types of 'others' who can be present during performance:

- An **audience** simply watches the play. Examples include the silent crowd at a snooker match or the chief scout from a local club making notes during a performance. The audience has no direct part in the performance but applies pressure simply by being there.
- **Supporters**, such as members of the crowd at a football match, are not content with simply watching; they are more interactive and cheer or criticise the performance. They can have a more direct bearing on the player since the encouragement they give can provide motivation.
- A **co-actor** is defined as someone doing the same activity without being in competition, like another jogger in the park when you are out for a run. Their mere presence may be an incentive to perform better.
- A **competitor** is in direct conflict with the performer, for example the other athletes in a 100m race. Competition in sport is a major cause of anxiety.

The main effect of being watched in sport is a rise in the performers' level of arousal. In the same way that arousal levels affect sports performers in different ways according to the inverted U theory, the effect of an audience can vary. An expert performer such as a

Key terms

Facilitation: a performance improved by external and internal influences.

Inhibition: a performance made worse by external and internal influences.

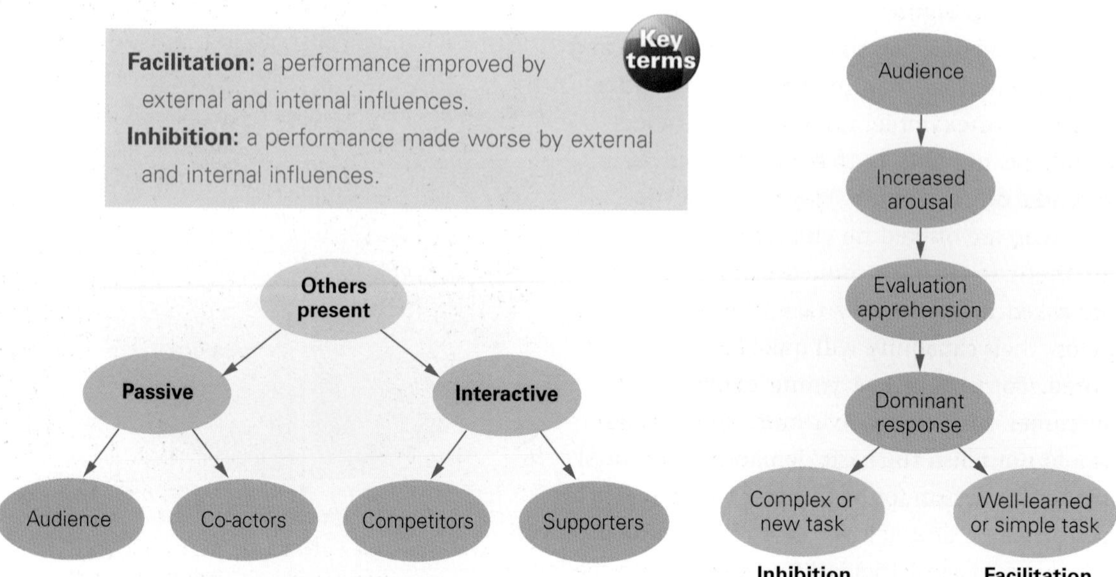

Figure 11.11 Four types of others during a performance

Figure 11.12 Social facilitation and social inhibition

professional football player will be used to playing in front of a crowd and will be able to cope with the pressure of being watched. Sometimes professional players raise their game for the big events and can respond to the crowd — we say their performance is **facilitated.** A novice performer will find the effect more daunting and may be put off by the presence of an audience, resulting in an **inhibited** performance.

The differing effects of an audience also relate to drive theory and the dominant response. At high arousal levels, the performer takes in less information from the environment and tends to focus on the dominant response. For experts who have learned the skill well this response is usually correct and so the performance is facilitated. Novices, however, may not yet have learned the correct response, so under pressure they choose the wrong options.

The type of task being performed is important in determining whether facilitation or inhibition takes place. A simple task requires less decision making and less information, so it can be performed correctly at high arousal levels. A complex task requires more decision making and may not be performed correctly at high levels of arousal when less information is processed by the performer. Therefore, a simple skill may be facilitated if an audience is present and a complex task may be inhibited.

An effect of being watched is a fear of being judged. **Evaluation apprehension** is the term used to describe the fear of being judged. Can you remember what it was like when your parents watched you in your first performance? You felt anxious not only because you were being watched for the first time, but also because you were a beginner. Years later, you might welcome your parents watching you play because as a more proficient player you are more confident. However, if the person watching you is an expert, such as a chief scout from a professional club, then although you know you can play well you still feel anxious about their presence.

The effects of being watched in sport can be influenced by the situation. Most players prefer to

Top tip

Questions on the effects of an audience may ask you to suggest two possible effects of being watched: inhibition or facilitation. Use Figure 11.12 to help you suggest that an audience can either make you perform better or worse. Think about increased arousal, evaluation apprehension and dominant response, then — depending on the performer of the task — how performance can be helped or hindered.

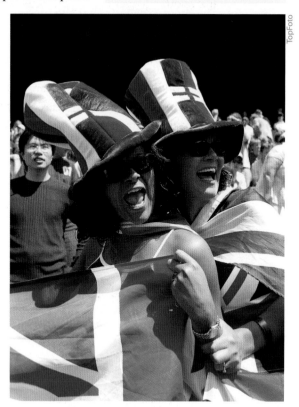

TopFoto

'Henmania' was often considered to be a contributing factor in Tim Henman's relatively poor showings at Wimbledon, despite his high world ranking

play on their home ground, in familiar surroundings, in front of a supportive crowd and such support can enhance performance. Playing away from home can be more distracting, especially when the away crowd is hostile. The preference for playing at home is called the 'home field advantage'. However, the expectation that a team will win at home can put undue pressure on the players and performance might be impaired.

Players who suffer from natural trait anxiety will be even more nervous in front of a big crowd. Remember that those who show trait anxiety are more likely to show state anxiety. Extrovert personalities are more likely to respond positively to the effects of an audience because they prefer to be loud and obvious in front of others. Introvert characters are more likely to suffer in front of an audience because they naturally wish to avoid the limelight. More experienced players are less likely to suffer from inhibition.

Distraction conflict theory

Have you ever been trying to watch an important game on television and been distracted by a member of your family asking you questions? It is hard to concentrate on two things at the same time. Distraction conflict explains why it is difficult to multi-task.

The theory suggests that the presence of a distraction, which may be from an external source such as the crowd, or from an internal source such as a worry about an injury, while the performer is trying to concentrate on the task will cause an increase in arousal levels. This, in turn, could cause performance to deteriorate, especially if the performer is a beginner. There is conflict between the demands of the task and the draw of the distraction. The effect of distractions is worse if the task is complex. If the distraction is intense, such as a loud shout from the crowd or from the opposition, then the effect can be immediate.

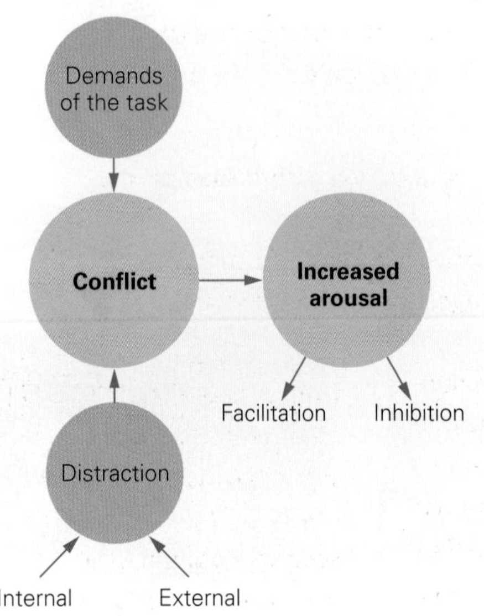

Figure 11.13 A summary of distraction conflict theory

There are methods that both the player and the coach can use to counter the effects of distraction and social inhibition and to promote social facilitation. A useful strategy is to allow the players to be watched when they train so that they get used to playing in front of a crowd. Parents and families could be invited to training and social events at the club. The coach could attempt to lower the perceived importance of the event. If a big league game is coming up, the coach could suggest that even if the game is lost there is still an opportunity to win the league.

The players could practise the techniques used to counter both somatic and cognitive anxieties. Relaxation techniques, visualisation and imagery, with special emphasis on games played in front of a big crowd, could be used to help reduce tension and lower levels of arousal.

In summary, playing in front of a crowd can have positive or negative effects depending on the complexity of the task and the experience of the players. Inhibition and facilitation can be explained by reference to the inverted U and drive theories, since the main effect of being watched is to increase arousal and these theories explain the relationship between arousal and performance.

Attribution theory

Key term

Attribute: to perceive a reason for an event, which can affect future effort and motivation.

Think of a major game or performance in which you did really well. What reasons can you give for your success? Was it due to your performance or due to things that were out of your control? Now think of a game in which you did not do so well. Were the reasons for that poor performance out of your control? If you listen to a summary of a game by two football managers after the final whistle you might realise that the reasons the winning manager gives for success are often different from those that the losing manager gives for failure.

Attribution theory looks at the reasons sports performers give for winning and losing.

According to Wiener's model, there are four main categories into which the reasons for winning and losing can be placed. The first two categories define the extent to which the performer has control over the outcome. They are known collectively as the **locus of causality**:

- An **internal reason** is one that is under the control or influence of the performer. Examples include the amount of effort put into the game, the level of ability shown during the performance and the amount of pre-performance practice.
- An **external reason** is one that is said to be outside the control of the performer. Examples include a decision given by a referee, the bounce of the ball or the quality of the opposing team.

The other two categories — collectively known as the **locus of stability** — define how permanent the perceived reasons for winning or losing are.

- A **stable reason** is one that takes time to change. The ability level of the performer is stable. This does not mean that the level of ability will never change, but it will take some time to improve.
- An **unstable reason** is one that is temporary and can change from moment to moment or from week to week. Unstable reasons include psychological factors (such as the impact of missing an open goal), task difficulty (such as playing against difficult opposition), luck (such as a ball hitting the crossbar and either deflecting in or out of the goal) and effort (such as a greater effort put in at the start of the season than at its close when the chances of winning the league have gone).

Key terms

Locus of causality: where the reasons for winning and losing are placed, either internally or externally.

Locus of stability: how permanent the reasons for winning and losing are.

Locus of causality

Locus of stability	Internal	External
Stable	**Ability**	**Coaching**
Unstable	**Effort** **Practice** **Psychological factors**	**Luck** **Task difficulty** **Teamwork** **Officials**

Figure 11.14 Wiener's model of attribution

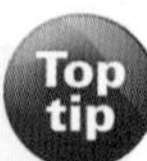

Make sure that you can give a sporting example for each attributional style.

Tasks to tackle 11.4

Make a copy of the matrix that shows the attributed reasons for success or failure. Consider the following reasons given by athletes for the outcome of a race in which they have just competed and place them in the appropriate area of the matrix:

(a) 'I was feeling good today and my performance reflected that feeling. I had the stamina to push right to the end.'

(b) 'I was given a poor draw in lane 8 and couldn't hear the starter, he just wasn't loud enough.'

(c) 'I gave it my all. I tried to keep up with the pace at the end and I was so nearly in the mix. In a few weeks I will be right up there with that lot, trust me!'

(d) 'We got our plan wrong. The coach suggested I push the pace early but maybe I did not push enough. It's back to the drawing board.'

The attribute of luck can therefore be classed as both unstable and external. The attribute of effort is both unstable and internal. We can sum up the reasons given for winning and losing on a matrix, as shown in Figure 11.14.

Self-serving bias

The tendency to blame losing on external and unstable reasons and account for victory using internal and stable reasons is called **self-serving bias**. Coaches can help to motivate players by blaming a loss on external influences beyond the athletes' control, such as bad luck or the decision of the referee. Success should be attributed to internal factors, such as the players' ability and efforts.

Coaches can use factors in the internal part of the attribution model (Figure 11.14) to motivate players, for example by rewarding effort, praising ability and criticising lack of effort.

Learned helplessness and mastery orientation

Learned helplessness is a state of mind that occurs when performers attribute losing to internal and stable reasons. Performers blame themselves and their own ability for losing and think that such failure is inevitable and likely to be repeated. Such learned helplessness can be specific to one sport, such as 'I just can't play tennis', or it can be more general — 'I'm no good at sport'. Causes of learned helplessness can be repeated failure, lack of encouragement from the coach or targets that are simply too high.

To counter learned helplessness the reasons for losing need to be changed from internal and stable ones to external and unstable ones, a process known as attributional retraining. Positive feedback and reinforcement should be offered to encourage more effort and reduce learned helplessness. The goals or targets should be changed, so that they are in line with the ability of the player. Improving the number of drop shots or successful service returns could be a goal that does not just include winning but stresses personal improvement. Such targets could be used to redefine failure in the sense that success is not just about winning but includes playing a better game despite the result.

Top tip

Attributions in sport are important to make sure that players keep motivated. Make sure that you can suggest ways to counter learned helplessness such as setting easy targets at first, being positive and rewarding and using self-serving bias — blaming external and unstable reasons for losing.

The opposite of learned helplessness is called mastery orientation. Players who show mastery orientation think that success can be repeated, that losing is temporary and can be overcome, and that the reasons for success are internal. Such players tend to show confidence and a real determination to keep on improving. They show the characteristics of a performer with the need to achieve and they are prepared to take risks and to take responsibility for their actions. Such players are just what the coach needs in the team to ensure that the reasons given for winning and losing are used to promote future effort.

Practice makes perfect

1. Goal setting is a strategy used by coaches to improve performance. Why should goal setting lead to improved performance and what principles should the coach consider when setting goals? *(6 marks)*
2. Name and explain the different forms of anxiety that might be experienced by a sports performer. *(4 marks)*
3. Some athletes tend to perform well when they are being watched, while others seem to choke under the pressure. Use your knowledge of psychological theories to explain the differing effects an audience can have on a performer. *(7 marks)*
4. After a competitive match, some players may give reasons for losing that generate feelings of learned helplessness. What is meant by the term learned helplessness and how can a coach prevent learned helplessness from happening? *(6 marks)*

Chapter 12 Evaluating contemporary influences

World Games and supporting the development of elite performers

What you need to know

By the end of this chapter you should be able to:

- understand the characteristics and impact of World Games
- describe the stages of Sport England's sport development continuum and the factors that influence performers' progression through it
- list and explain the social and cultural factors required to support performers' progression from the participation stage to the performance and excellence stages
- explain the role and structure of the World Class Performance Pathway in funding elite performers
- explain the roles and purposes of key organisations in supporting and progressing performers from grass roots to elite levels

Key characteristics of World Games

Global sporting events, also known as World Games, can be identified by a number of key features:

- They attract the best **elite** performers in the world with the aim of deciding the world's number 1.
- There is a high level of commercialisation linked to worldwide media coverage.
- They may be multi-sport (such as the Olympic Games) or feature a single sport (such as the football World Cup).
- They present a chance to bring nations together in a sporting festival atmosphere.

Key terms

World Games: multi-sport or single-sport global events that bring together the top-class elite performers of the world, for example the Olympic Games, the football World Cup.

Elite: describes excellence-level performers, for example those capable of performing for their country at World Games events.

Top tip

It should be noted that the characteristics of World Games apply to high-profile sports only, such as football and athletics. Minority sports may have the best performers striving to be number 1 in the world, but they receive little media coverage, with a resultant loss of sponsorship and financial gain. The World Trampolining Championships, for example, cannot be described as a World Games.

- They give a chance to promote 'nation building' — to develop national pride by showing a country in its best light by hosting the event and/or being successful in it. A good example of nation building was seen in Beijing, China throughout the Olympic Games of 2008.
- Deviancy, such as drug taking and cheating, may result.

The impact of World Games events

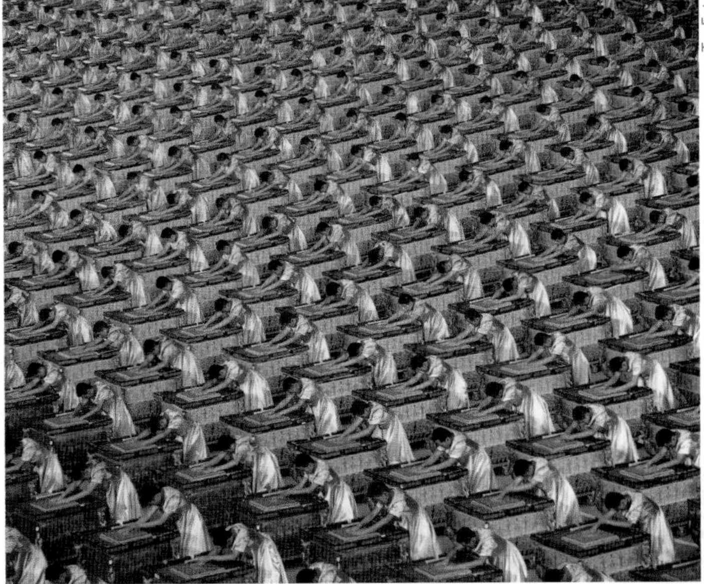
TopFoto

Performers at the Olympic opening ceremony in Beijing. The ceremony provides the opportunity to showcase the host nation to the rest of the world.

During 2007–08, the estimated cost of staging the London 2012 Olympics reached over £9 billion as projected planning and building costs were reported in the media. Even the process of bidding to host a World Games is expensive and time consuming. Why do nations such as the UK bid to host global sporting events when the costs are so great?

The advantages listed in Table 12.1 on p. 114 can be seen to impact at the level of individual members of the public. Many people live in areas designated to benefit from the legacy of 2012. The Lea Valley Olympic precinct, for example, will include a main stadium and other key sporting venues such as an aquatics centre, a velodrome and three indoor arenas. The construction of the Olympic Village necessitates improvements to surrounding infrastructure such as bridges, underpasses and existing waterways.

> **Top tip**
> The infrastructure of Athens benefited from hosting the 2004 Olympics with a new international airport, an expanded metro system and an ultra-modern traffic management centre.

In addition, the investment of billions of pounds into elite sports events impacts at the level of the individual athletes. World Games:

- give an opportunity for some athletes to represent their country on 'home soil'
- give an opportunity to perform at the highest level and seek recognition as the 'best in the world'
- provide an opportunity to develop friendships in a spirit of friendly sporting rivalry (i.e. social integration)
- establish the performer's name and possibly offer extrinsic rewards, such as sponsorship opportunities, as a result of success

Chapter 12 World Games and supporting the development of elite performers

Table 12.1 Advantages and disadvantages of staging a World Games for the host nation

Advantages	Disadvantages
International promotion of the host city and country Social inclusion/integration and improved cultural relationships both within the host nation and internationally Regeneration through improvements to infrastructure, such as transport links, as well as the legacy of sports facilities, athlete accommodation blocks, and so on An increase in national pride — the feel-good factor of hosting a World Games leads to success by some national performers Economic benefits of tourism Health and fitness benefits as the nation responds to positive role models	Relocation of home owners and businesses to accommodate infrastructure developments High costs to taxpayers and the diversion of funds from other areas of society The possibility of national debt if not commercially successful Threat from terrorists Overcrowding and disruption to everyday life Legacy of unused facilities left after the Games if this is not thought through at the planning stage

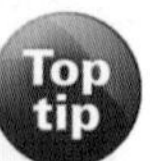

See **www.sportengland.org/2012_uk** for benefits of the 2012 Olympics to the UK.

Tasks to tackle 12.1

Discuss the following statement: 'Hosting the 2012 Olympic Games will be nothing but beneficial for the people of the UK.'

Sport England's sport development continuum

During your AS studies, the sports development continuum may have been introduced as the **performance pyramid**. The first stage of the continuum is called the foundation stage, proceeding through participation and performance to excellence, as illustrated in Figure 12.1.

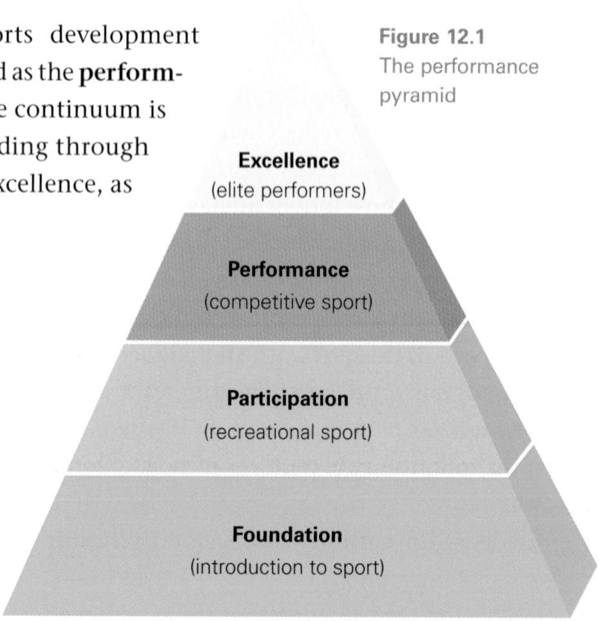

Key term

Performance pyramid: a model that illustrates the progressive development of an athlete from beginner (i.e. foundation stage) to elite level (i.e. excellence stage).

Excellence (elite performers)

Performance (competitive sport)

Participation (recreational sport)

Foundation (introduction to sport)

Figure 12.1 The performance pyramid

Factors influencing the progression to sports excellence

One of the first steps in achieving sports excellence is to discover the potential talent in the first place. When looking to discover potential talent (perhaps at the performance level) a number of qualities may be looked for.

> **Top tip**
> In this section of A2, the focus is on elite-level performers who have reached national and international standards of performance as well as achieving other characteristics required in the modern-day sporting world to progress them through various stages of the continuum.

Physical qualities may include an individual's natural ability, pain threshold, fitness levels and their somatotype or body type. Sporting Giants, for example, is a UK Sport initiative that identifies performers with height as an initial physical quality necessary for rowing, basketball, volleyball etc.

Psychological qualities may include being highly competitive, mentally tough and highly motivated. Successful sports performers need to be able to deal with constructive criticism, to control internal arousal levels, and be willing to train and make sacrifices in the long term in order to be successful.

Social and cultural factors also impact on sports progression and can be influential, even at school level, in determining which sport an individual will initially participate in as well as possible progression to elite levels. Social and cultural influences include:

- a tradition of sports participation
- parental influence, family support, religious preferences
- popularity of sport at school
- teachers' specialities and interests
- positive role models and the impact of media coverage
- accessible facilities for different activities in the local area
- structured levels of competition
- availability of specialist coaching

There is an important link between the participation stage and the excellence stage of the participation pyramid: the larger the base of participation, the more likely it is that a greater number of athletes will filter towards the top. Therefore, it is important that the base of talent identification is as wide as possible. In addition, sports themselves need to become more open and democratic by reducing the incidence of discrimination, be it racial, sexual or class-based.

> **Top tip**
> It is important that you develop an understanding of different factors that determine whether a person will reach elite level in his/her sport. In relation to elite performers, all contributing factors — facilities, coaches, skills — need to be high level, as opposed to just 'good'.

Talent identification and development programmes

Working in partnership, UK Sport, the English Institute of Sport (EIS) and national governing Bodies (NGBs) of sport are committed to systematically unearthing sporting talent with the necessary skills and mindset to win medals and world titles in a few years' time.

Wherever they take place, **talent identification** and development programmes need to consider:

- physiological factors, such as fitness measurements
- **anthropometry**, such as height in volleyball etc.
- psychological factors, such as mental toughness
- hereditary factors, or natural 'advantages'
- sociological and cultural factors, such as family support

Key terms

Talent identification: a process by which children are encouraged to participate in the sports at which they are most likely to succeed. It is based on testing certain 'parameters' that are designed to predict performance capacity, taking into account the child's current level of fitness and maturity.

Anthropometry: the scientific measurement of the human body.

Talent identification and development programmes should be planned and organised to meet the needs of various sports and different age groups. Successful programmes will ensure a wide foundation and move performers along the continuum towards excellence by:

- screening all potential performers
- directing performers to sports most suited to their talents
- giving the chance to accelerate the developmental process
- providing efficient use of the funding available — offering funds at different stages of the athlete's development
- offering access to specialist facilities and services, such as physiotherapy and performance lifestyle support (see pages 126–27), to support progression
- offering well-structured competitive programmes at various performance levels
- providing a coordinated approach between organisations — administration, record keeping and the division of roles should all be clear
- monitoring their own provision to build on good practice

However, talent identification programmes may have some drawbacks. They may miss 'late developers', they are viewed by some critics as expensive, and they give no guarantee of success.

Organisational support structure

All the organisations involved in sport aim to ensure smooth and seamless pathways that release the sporting potential in as many people as possible, including volunteers, coaches, officials, and the athletes themselves.

Table 12.2 Summary of sporting organisations

Support provided	By whom?
Financial support and investment	National governing bodies SportsAid Sponsorship National Lottery UK Sport Sport England
High-quality coaching and specialist, top-level facilities	English Institute of Sport (EIS) UK Institute of Sport Sports Coach UK National governing bodies Centres of excellence UK Sport Sport England
Sports science (technology, physiotherapy, medicine, nutrition)	English Institute of Sport (EIS) Centres of excellence National governing bodies Higher education institutions (as part of EIS)
Talent identification	National governing bodies UK Sport (2012 talent identification initiatives, e.g. Girls4Gold, Pitch2Podium, Sporting Giants, Sprint Kayak) EIS regional scouts Sport England
Structured, progressive levels of competition and training in elite groups	Academies Centres of excellence Specialist schools, sports colleges County and regional squads, development squads Training camps

Top tip

In the exam you can only be asked direct questions on organisations and initiatives actually included in the specification, so your focus should be on these.

It is important to understand the main aims and policies of the organisations listed in the specification as opposed to their actual structure.

Sport England

Sport England is the government agency responsible for developing a world-class community sports system. In June 2008, Sport England published a new strategy designed to get more people playing and enjoying sport, as well as helping those with talent to get to the very top. This strategy committed Sport England to working with national governing bodies and local authorities to deliver three clear objectives:

- **Grow** — increasing participation. Approximately 15% of Sport England's investment will be focused on increasing regular participation in sport by 200 000 per year. The target is to get 1 million additional individuals doing more sport by 2012–13, for example via the 'free swimming' initiative for the under 16s and over 60s. This target will be measured through the Active People surveys. In addition to this, working in partnership with the Youth Sport Trust, Sport England will help more young people gain access to 5 hours of sport a week.
- **Sustain** — decreasing the 'drop out' and increasing participant satisfaction. Approximately 60% of Sport England's investment will focus on sustaining current participation in sport by seeking to ensure a high-quality sporting experience, particularly with respect to the 16–18 age group where the 'drop off' has been traditionally high when PE is no longer compulsory. The target for 2012–13 is to decrease by 25% the number of 16-year-olds who drop out of sport in five key sports. Sport England will aim to increase the satisfaction of sports participants through high-quality experiences.
- **Excel** — increase talent. Approximately 25% of Sport England's investment will focus on developing and accelerating talent identification and support systems for different sports. In partnerships with NGBs, a key aim will be to ensure talented individuals receive the right level of coaching provision at appropriate levels.

Top tip

Sport England does not build facilities but it does improve facilities for sport by investing Lottery funds in them.

Sport England, NGBs and Whole Sport Plans (WSPs)

In 2003, Sport England identified 30 priority sports, based on their capability to contribute to Sport England's vision of an active and successful sporting nation. Sport England continues to work with the NGBs of these sports to assist in the development and implementation of their Whole Sport Plan (WSP).

What are WSPs?

Each WSP looks at the whole of a sport from grass roots through to elite level and identifies how it will achieve its vision and contribute to Sport England's 'grow', 'sustain' and 'excel' objectives.

The plans identify the help and resources NGBs need in order to deliver their vision. They therefore assist Sport England in directing funding and resources to NGBs. They also provide measurable targets against which Sport England can assess the NGBs' achievements and value for money. Importantly, WSPs also help to create links between the different regions of the UK and the different partners involved in all aspects of sport.

From mid-2008 onwards, NGBs were required to develop their WSPs to illustrate how they proposed to deliver against the 'grow', 'sustain' and 'excel' targets (such as decreasing drop out by 25%). These WSPs will be regularly assessed and reviewed by Sport England, with NGBs being given a single grant lasting 4 years to deliver their stated aims. The aim of this single grant is to cut down on bureaucracy by providing money from a single pot, as opposed to different funding streams.

An important part of the WSPs will be the provision of coaches to develop talent (excel), improve satisfaction (sustain) and encourage participation (grow). The Youth Sport Trust and NGBs will work with Sport England to develop a 'Coaching for Young People' strand linked to delivering the 'Five Hour Sports Offer'.

Links with the Youth Sport Trust and UK Sport

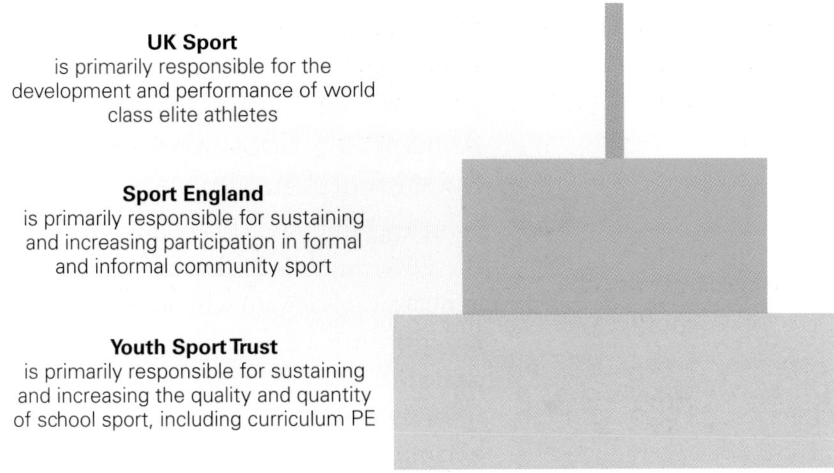

UK Sport
is primarily responsible for the development and performance of world class elite athletes
Sport England
is primarily responsible for sustaining and increasing participation in formal and informal community sport
Youth Sport Trust
is primarily responsible for sustaining and increasing the quality and quantity of school sport, including curriculum PE

Figure 12.2 The relationship between UK Sport, Sport England and the Youth Sport Trust

Historically, the transition from school sport to elite-level sport has not always been as smooth as any of the associated organisations would have wanted. This is shown by the massive decline in sport participation that occurs at 16 (the post-school gap discussed at AS), and the difficulties some elite athletes from more deprived backgrounds face in getting to the podium. In order to make the transition from school sport to community sport smoother, Sport England needs to reach down into the Youth Sport Trust area to run alongside them ahead of the handover at 16. Sport England's role in this area is to ensure, through its work with sports nationally, regionally and locally, that the sporting environment is attractive and supportive of young people. This will help to ensure they stay in sport once they leave compulsory schooling. Sport England attempts to ensure this through:

- club development — ensuring clubs are strong enough to reach out to schools and young people
- community sports provision — including non-sports youth clubs such as the Scouts
- helping NGBs develop effective competition frameworks for children and young people
- the development of NGB volunteering strategies for young people

Sport England therefore has a crucial role to play in ensuring the success of the 'Five Hour Sports Offer' for children and young people, It is also involved in the 'Sport Unlimited' initiative offering 10-week taster sessions in sports children have requested in the hope they will continue their sporting involvement when the 10 weeks are up. Other projects include the 'Step into Sport', 'School Club Links' and 'Extending Activities' initiatives.

Sport England also has an important role to play in reaching up and linking with UK Sport's World Class Performance Programme. For this to succeed, its investment in NGBs requires comprehensive and effective athlete pathways from clubs through to World Class Performance Programmes. Sport England is responsible for funding elite sport for non-Olympic sports such as squash and netball. It also funds the Commonwealth Games Council of England. In reality, Sport England sees such links to elite sport as 'a modest element' of its role and remit.

Top tip

To find out more information about the new kitemarks see: **www.teachernet.gov.uk/pe**

Tasks to tackle 12.2

Give three policies Sport England has developed to encourage increased participation in sport and broaden the base from which to develop talent.

Activemark, Sportsmark and Sports Partnership Mark

Sport England was actively involved in establishing the government's PE kitemark programme. These annual awards reward schools in their delivery of the government's PE School Sport and Young People strategy (PESSYP). Schools need to meet a number of set criteria. Only schools within a school sport partnership are eligible and the kitemarks are awarded through the National School Sport Survey, which all partnership schools take part in. Successful schools are awarded a certificate and are allowed to use the kitemark logo for the 1-year duration of the award.

Other home country sports councils

The Sports Council for Wales is the national organisation responsible for developing and promoting sport and active lifestyles in Wales. It is the main adviser on sporting matters to the Welsh Assembly Government and is responsible for distributing funds from the National Lottery to sport in Wales. The main themes of the Council's work are active young people, active communities and developing performance and excellence. The Council fully subscribes to the Welsh Assembly Government's vision for a physically active and sporting nation, as outlined in its strategy document 'Climbing Higher'. To support 'Climbing Higher', the Council has published a Framework for the Development of Sport and Physical Activity. The Framework commits the Sports Council for Wales to a shift from grants management to sports development through the marketing of physical activity, advocacy for sport and innovation in programme development.

Sport Scotland is the national agency for sport in Scotland. Its mission is to encourage everyone in Scotland to discover and develop their own sporting experience, helping to increase participation and improve performances in Scottish sport. Through a trust company it operates three National Centres providing quality, affordable, residential and sporting facilities and services for the development of people in sport. Sport Scotland is also the parent company of the Scottish Institute of Sport (see page 129).

Sport Northern Ireland is committed to 'Making Sport Happen' for as many people as possible. It is committed to working with its partners to:

- increase and sustain committed participation, especially among young people
- raise the standards of sporting excellence and promote the good reputation and efficient administration of sport
- support individuals working in sport from administrators and coaches/leaders through to officials, so that as many people as possible can get involved in physical activity

Its schemes include the Junior Club Development Pack (underpinning club development), Running Sport courses (improving club management and administration) and the Sport for All leader award scheme (training community-based sports leaders).

UK Sport

Established by Royal Charter in 1996, UK Sport works in partnership with the home country sports councils and other agencies to lead sport in the UK to world-class success. UK Sport is responsible for managing and distributing public investment and distributes funds raised by the National Lottery. It is accountable to Parliament through the Department for Culture, Media and Sport.

It takes around 8 years for athletes to reach their peak once their talent has been identified and nurtured. This process involves support providers from top-level coaches and physiotherapists to doctors and biomechanists. Nothing can be left to chance, from the kit the athletes use to the food they eat and the tactics their coaches employ. UK Sport's mission is to support the delivery necessary for success at the world's most significant sporting events — principally the Olympic and Paralympic Games.

Key term

UK Sport: an organisation that focuses on the support and development of elite-level athletes in the UK.

Top tip

For up-to-date information on the work of UK Sport in relation to elite sport, and a free newsletter, visit **www.uksport.gov.uk**.

Key term

World Class Performance Programme: an initiative designed to support elite-level athletes with funding to enable full-time training.

World Class Performance Programme

Winning medals on the international sporting stage is hard and the margins between success and failure become smaller every year. To ensure that the UK's most talented athletes have the chance to realise their potential, UK Sport has created the **World Class Performance Programme**.

UK Sport now funds athletes via NGB recommendations through one of three distinct World Class Pathways:

- **Podium** — this pathway supports athletes with realistic medal capabilities at the next Olympic or Paralympic Games (i.e. a maximum of 4 years away from the podium).
- **Development** — this supports athletes who have demonstrated realistic medal capabilities (typically 6 years away from the podium).
- **Talent** — this supports identification and confirmation of athletes who have the potential to progress to a higher pathway with the help of targeted investment (typically 8 years away from the podium).

Having run the programme since 1997 and with the benefit of lessons learned from the Sydney and Athens Olympics, UK Sport has developed a **no compromise** approach to funding and support. Its investment strategy targets resources at athletes capable of delivering medal-winning performances. Individual sports are allocated funding based on a combination of past performance and future potential.

> Key term
> **No compromise:** this ultimately means taking no short cuts in resourcing the best athletes to realise their medal ambitions.

Some 1500 of the nation's leading athletes at the podium and development levels alone benefit from an annual investment of £100 million (comprising both National Lottery and Government Exchequer funds), with many more involved at the talent level. The programme delivers funds by two channels:

- sport performance programmes via NGBs
- individual, means-tested Athlete Personal Awards

Each sport's Performance Programme is overseen by a performance director, and could include any (or all) of the following:

- world class coaches
- sports science and medicine support
- warm weather training and acclimatisation
- international competition schedule
- athlete development programmes
- access to appropriate training facilities

This support is worth around £55 000 per athlete per annum at the podium level and £30 000 per athlete at the development stage, depending on the sport.

In addition, all athletes are entitled to apply for an Athlete Personal Award (APA). This is paid directly to the athlete and contributes to their living costs and their personal sporting costs.

The level of APA received is determined by a number of criteria, including which Performance Pathway the athlete is on. While there are variations depending on the sport, three performance categories apply for podium athletes:

- Band A — medallist at Olympic or World Championship level; maximum award £23 930
- Band B — top eight finish at Olympic or world level competition; maximum award £17 948
- Band C — likely to be a major championship performer, but flexibility given to individual sports to set their own criteria; maximum award £11 965

The average APA payment to athletes on the podium programme is currently around £17 000. The average figure for development level athletes is closer to £7000. Funding is awarded on the basis of an Olympic cycle and commences on 1 April in the year immediately following a Games, for a period of 4 years.

Top tip

In questions relating to sports excellence you need to link raising standards to receiving top-quality coaching, facilities and equipment. Do not just write 'more' facilities, 'better' coaching etc., as this will not earn marks.

Tasks to tackle 12.3

Place the following eight sports in descending order of amounts received from the World Class Performance Programme 2006–09 before the Beijing Olympics (i.e. highest amount at the top).

Weightlifting Athletics Swimming Rowing Hockey Triathlon Table tennis Cycling

1 ....

2 ....

3 ....

4 ....

5 ....

6 ....

7 ....

8 ....

Make an 'educated guess' first, then visit the UK Sport website and visit the pages for summer Olympic sports.

World Class Events Programme

UK Sport leads the campaign to bring strategically important sporting events to Britain. Working in partnership with NGBs, cities and regions and home country sports councils,

UK Sport coordinates the UK's efforts to bid for and stage major events. Since 1997, UK Sport has supported more than 120 events of world, European and Commonwealth status. It expects that the build-up to 2012 will increase the impetus to bid for and stage world-class events.

Through the National Lottery-funded World Class Events Programme, UK Sport is investing some £20 million into UK-hosted events between 2006 and 2012 and has identified 28 World Championships and 27 European Championships that it hopes to bid for and stage over the next few years. In 2008, UK Sport supported 17 events, including a record six World Championships.

In addition to the World Class Events Programme, UK Sport acts as the strategic lead in events research, capacity building and knowledge transfer. Ahead of London 2012, capacity building is especially crucial. With a target of ensuring that at least 65% of officials are British, staging major events on home soil is a prime opportunity for officials to gain the necessary experience and to equip personnel with key skills.

In 2006, UK Sport established an Event Managers Education and Development Programme for event organisers from UK NGBs. The programme provides a forum for harnessing and transferring knowledge between sports and sharing best practice.

A good example of the success of the World Class Events Programme was seen at the 2008 UCI World Track Cycling Championships which were held in March. The British team swept the board, winning 50% of the gold medals available. Chris Hoy, who won two golds and a silver at the championships, commented on the significance of competing at home to the successes achieved.

In considering world-class events, UK Sport's events team considers not only likely performance impact, but also the broader impacts of issues such as the wider sporting, social, cultural, economic and environmental benefits and likely legacy.

Mission 2012

Mission 2012 is UK Sport's project designed to keep eyes focused on every aspect of the performance system in the build-up to the London Olympics. The project encourages sports to conduct their own assessments of how their system is performing and to bring additional expertise to bear in finding creative solutions to problems. Both good practice and potential problems will be tracked over the remaining years ahead of the 2012 Games.

Mission 2012 requires sports to think about their performance plans based around:

- athletes' performance and development
- the performance system
- the leadership and climate that exist within the sport

Sports' assessments are reviewed every quarter by two special Mission 2012 panels (one for Olympic sports and one for Paralympic sports), consisting of Steve Cram, Sir Clive Woodward and Rod Carr (Olympic panel) and Dame Tanni Grey-Thompson, Sue Wolstenholme and

Chris Holmes (Paralympic panel). The panels consider the suitability of proposed action plans and examine other areas where they think they can add value.

Promoting 'ethically fair, drug-free' sport

UK Sport's Sporting Conduct initiative is aimed at improving fair play in the competitive sporting arena. It is also responsible for the implementation and management of the UK's anti-doping policy. In 2006, nearly 8000 tests across 50 different sports were carried out, with results published quarterly on the UK Sport website. In May 2005, UK Sport started its '100% Me' campaign. This is designed to provide a platform for athletes to celebrate their success in drug-free competition and as drug-free competitors and to provide positive role models to future generations.

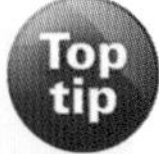

To test your knowledge of drug-free sport go to: **www.100percentme.co.uk/home.php**

Working in partnership

In July 2007, UK Sport and SportsAid, the sports charity, revealed a new partnership designed to support emerging athletes across 35 sports in the build-up to the London Olympics and Paralympics in 2012. The partnership is a result of changes to the Talented Athlete Scholarship Scheme (TASS) introduced to clarify the way in which the scholarships are awarded. Since TASS, and its sister programme TASS 2012, was introduced in 2004 more than 3000 athletes have received financial support, helping them to maximise their sporting potential without compromising their academic careers. From April 2008, UK Sport announced that it will allocate £8 million of TASS funding to athletes in summer Olympic sports over a 4-year cycle through to London 2012. This money will be part of the overall funding package for NGBs, designed to maximise medal opportunities at the London Games. A further £12 million will be administered by SportsAid in the same period to TASS and TASS 2012 athletes outside of those summer Olympic sports.

Elite sport support services

Coaching, sports science and medicine, lifestyle support and research all play an important role in ensuring the ongoing success of British athletes.

Coaching

The UK Sport coaching team aims to deliver quality coaching to athletes on UK Sport's World Class Performance Pathway. To achieve this, the UK Sport World Class Coaching Strategy must deliver targeted and innovative programmes specific to the needs of world-class coaches. The strategy has three key elements:

- **World Class Coaching Conference.** Since its inception in 2001, the World Class Coaching Conference has been established as an annual event and a must for coaches in all high-performance sports. The conference provides a forum for the best coaches in the UK to meet, debate and share best practice. The aim is to equip coaches with the skills and knowledge to make sustainable changes to an athlete's training programme. The best national and international speakers are sought to present to over 350 coaches working with British athletes.

- **Elite Coach.** Launched after the Athens Olympics in 2004, Elite Coach is a 3-year accelerated coach development programme in which up to ten coaches per year are selected to participate. Elite Coach is a targeted, focused and fully supported programme for the best coaches who demonstrate the talent, dedication and determination to succeed and produce outstanding performances.
- **Winning Coaches.** This programme is further divided in three:
  - The Workshop Programme is a series of multi-sport workshops developed specifically for high-performance coaches in the UK. These are designed to address current issues and needs of the coach and introduce new developments. They also offer opportunities to deliver solutions to issues arising from Mission 2012.
  - The Coaching Team Programme focuses on coaching, training and evaluating the work of high-performance teams.
  - The Podium Coaches Programme is targeted at coaches who led athletes, teams and sports in Beijing 2008. It aims to continue their work into the lead-up to 2012.

Themes covered in the above programmes include managing relationships, neuro-linguistic programming, time management, team start-up and decision making.

Sports medicine and sports science

UK Sport's sports medicine and sports science team works with partner organisations to continually challenge and improve the level of scientific and medical support provided to the UK's elite athletes leading up to 2012 and beyond. It focuses on the following:

- **Evolution** — the continual strive to find better ways of supporting, delivering and improving sport medicine and sport science practice in the UK.
- **Professional development** — creating professional development programmes for the UK's sports medicine and sports science practitioners. The programmes utilise input from the UK's university sector, sports medicine and sports science associations, and leading sports medicine and sports science practitioners from the UK and the rest of the world.
- **Provision** — providing practitioners with access to services that will facilitate their performance impact. For example, all full-time NGB and home country sports council practitioners have been given membership to the Royal Society of Medicine, which allows access to library services. In 2008–09 a website was introduced by UK Sport's sports medicine and sports science team, to help give practitioners access to information and an opportunity to share best practice.

Performance Lifestyle

Elite athletes have to fit many aspects of their life into their intensive training programme. Performance Lifestyle is an individualised support service specifically designed to help each athlete create the unique environment necessary for his/her success. The approach is to work closely with coaches and support specialists as part of an integrated team to minimise potential concerns, conflicts and distractions, all of which can be detrimental to performance and, at worst, may end a career prematurely.

Lifestyle support is available on:

- time management
- budgeting and finance
- dealing with the media
- sponsorship and promotion activities
- negotiation/conflict management

Careers and employment advice is available on

- finding a job to supplement income and fit around training demands
- finding work placements to give a taste of possible careers options
- planning for a second career after sport

UK Sport's advisers have links with local employers and the **OPEN** programme to promote the range of skills and experience athletes can bring to the workplace.

Key terms

Olympic and Paralympic Employment Network (OPEN): the British Olympic Association's programme for finding employment for athletes.

Innovation Partners: an organisation or individual recognised by UK Sport as providing services that meet the world class standards of excellence in performance science and innovation required to make an impact on the UK's best athletes and coaches.

Research and innovation

UK Sport's research and innovation team works to encourage the generation of novel ideas and methods. It hopes to reach everyone with a passion for innovation in elite sport, from the highest level of expertise within its **Innovation Partner** network, to amateur enthusiasts and students through the Ideas 4 Innovation programme. Example innovation partners include BAE Systems (a global defence and aerospace company) and Loughborough University Sports Technology Institute.

The hunt for London 2012 talent

In partnership with the English Institute of Sport (EIS) and targeted national governing bodies, UK Sport is committed to systematically unearthing athletic talent, leading to possible participation in specialist fast-track programmes towards London 2012. UK Sport's talent identification programmes are highly scientific, involving a series of rigorous assessments and filters to detect individuals who have a higher probability of podium success. The system has to be smart enough to select individuals based on their future abilities and the standards required to deliver medals in a relatively short time. On average it takes 6–8 years for a promising sportsman or woman to get to the point at which he/she can deliver medals on the world's senior stage — but 2012 is nearer than that! UK Sport has undertaken a number of special talent identification initiatives, as detailed below.

Girls4Gold

This programme searches for highly competitive sportswomen with the potential to become Olympic champions in cycling and other targeted Olympic sports (e.g. canoeing, modern pentathlon, rowing and sailing) in time for London 2012. Girls4Gold is the most extensive female sporting talent recruitment drive ever undertaken in Great Britain. The ultimate aim of Girls4Gold is to unearth exceptional female talent capable of achieving medal success in London in 2012.

Pitch2Podium

This programme was created by UK Sport, the English Institute of Sport (EIS) and partners within the football authorities. Its aim is to provide young footballers who have been unsuccessful in securing a professional football contract with a second opportunity to succeed via the Olympics. Such players will have acquired some excellent skills, abilities and athletic qualities from their time in football. With elite coaching and the right support package, many of these attributes could be successfully switched to targeted Olympic sports, where they could achieve Olympic success in 2012.

Sporting Giants

In February 2007, UK Sport asked potential athletes to make themselves known, providing they fulfilled the basic criteria of being tall (a minimum of 6'3" or 190 cm for men and 5'11" or 180 cm for women), young (between 16 and 25) and with some sort of athletic background. The incentive was the potential for the most talented to become part of the performance programme in the Olympic sports of handball, rowing or volleyball.

Sprint Kayak

Flat water canoeing is a multi-medal sport at the Olympic Games. The GB Canoeing Programme, in partnership with UK Sport and the EIS, is focused on a nationwide search to assemble a highly competitive K4 crew. UK Sport has focused its search on 'ready-made' athletes who can transfer from 'like' sports, such as retired swimmers (or swimmers nearing retirement), to undertake a specialist fast-track Olympic Development Programme towards medal success in London 2012.

UK Sports Institute (UKSI)

In the spring of 1999, UK Sport, the four home country sports councils and the Department for Media, Culture and Sport, initiated the formation of the UKSI network. This consists of ten regional centres in England, with separate national centres in Scotland, Wales and Northern Ireland. The UKSI network has been important in the establishment of world-class facilities for top performers to train and compete in. Programmes of excellence across the UK are coordinated at UKSI headquarters in London. The UKSI's main role is to monitor and assess the quality of the service and facilities offered to sports and athletes across the network. The UKSI also coordinates research and development, drawing upon best practice from across the world and applying this to UK sports and excellence-level athletes.

UKSI national network centres

In practice, the network centres, such as Crystal Palace (South East) and the University of Bath (South West), act as a coordinating mechanism to harness the services in the region in which they are situated. UKSI Scotland is based at the University of Sterling, while UKSI Northern Ireland is based at the University of Ulster. In Wales, the UKSI is based at the Welsh Institute of Sport in Cardiff.

The primary role of each network centre is to assist NGBs and their top performers, as identified through the World Class Programme, to reach their targets in terms of world championships and medals. The network centres therefore provide the best sports coaches, high-quality facilities, equipment, sports scientists, medical professionals and various support personnel (such as lifestyle advisors) for elite athletes attending them. They also act as a vehicle for accessing an overseas network of facilities, including warm weather training, acclimatisation, altitude training and winter sports venues. Athletes selected to receive institute support have tailor-made programmes to help them develop as world-class athletes.

The **English Institute of Sport** (EIS) supports sports performers working at the highest level, or those who have the potential to do so. It is a nationwide network of centres throughout England that have various specialisms. For example, the centre at Loughborough specialises in athletics. At a regional level, the institutes of sport offer a range of mandatory services to give generic sports science and sports medicine support, such as acclimatisation, physical conditioning, sports massage and physiotherapy. Links are made with staff in facilities throughout each region to ensure a coordinated sports programme accessing the best coaches, equipment and facilities. To ensure educational and employment options are understood, links are also made to appropriate establishments in the areas served, as well as giving performance lifestyle advice.

Key term

English Institute of Sport: a network of world-class support services designed to develop the talents of elite athletes in England.

The **Scottish Institute of Sport** was set up by Sport Scotland in 1998. It is funded by the Sport Scotland Lottery fund and caters for over 200 athletes from a wide variety of sports. The University of Stirling became its main site in the autumn of 2002, offering a purpose-built facility acting as a hub for a network of six other centres, each of which is responsible for identifying and nurturing sports talent in its own region. In addition, the Scottish institutes and the area institutes form part of the UK-wide network, thus ensuring that Scottish athletes have access to the best support, wherever in the UK they are based.

UKSI-Cymru is a network of services offered to athletes in Wales and is coordinated by the Sports Council for Wales. It also provides athletes with world-class facilities, sports science, sports medicine and lifestyle support. As elsewhere in the UK, the institute operates a network of sites with the Welsh Institute of Sport, based at Sophia Gardens in Cardiff, acting as the hub.

Sports Institute Northern Ireland (SINI) is based at Jordanstown and is a partnership between the Sports Council for Northern Ireland and the University of Ulster. SINI aims to provide specialist services and key facilities for over 100 able-bodied and disabled national and international sportsmen and women to improve their competitive capability. Services provided are similar to the other home country institutes and include access to top-level coaches, training facilities, sports medicine, sports science and performance lifestyle advice.

Top tip

You can find out more about the work of each institute on the home country websites:t
www.sportengland.org.uk
www.sportscotland.org.uk
www.sports-council-wales.co.uk
www.sportscouncil-ni.org.uk

Tasks to tackle 12.4

Identify ways in which UK Sport influences sports excellence in the UK.

National governing bodies of sport

National governing bodies (NGBs) of sport such as UK Athletics and British Swimming have various responsibilities to fulfil. They maintain the rules and discipline of their sport and promote their sport throughout the UK and internationally. To continue to receive UK Sport Lottery funding, and to attract sponsorship and media deals, they must put in place initiatives to try to ensure success at international sporting events such as the Olympics. Some of the ways NGBs try to improve sports excellence include:

- maintaining talent identification schemes
- providing financial support, such as Athlete Personal Awards
- selection and recommendation of athletes for World Class Performance funding, SportsAid, TASS funding
- access to high-level facilities and equipment
- training high-level coaches and establishing specialist development squads
- providing sports science and medical support
- organising and providing information about competitions at different levels
- providing lifestyle advice and mentors
- working in partnership with other organisations, such as UK Sport and the British Olympic Association

Long Term Athlete Development (LTAD)

Long Term Athlete Development (LTAD) involves NGBs putting in place a structure that helps to prepare and encourage lifelong involvement in sport. Some common principles of player/performer development have been identified and then applied by NGBs as appropriate to their sport and the aspirations of participants in that sport, be they recreational or elite. LTAD establishes its role at the earliest opportunity, preparing youngsters for healthy lifelong participation in sport.

The LTAD pathway involves the progressions shown in Figure 12.3.

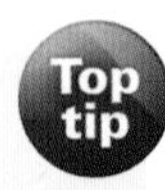

See **www.theFA.com** for the FA's Long Term Performer Development model.

Top tip

Sports excellence questions may relate to specific organisations (such as UK Sport) and their functions, or may require you to link together what you know about a number of different organisations (such as UK Sport, SportsAid and NGBs) in relation to 'winning more medals'. Whatever is asked for, try to make relevant points that answer the question set.

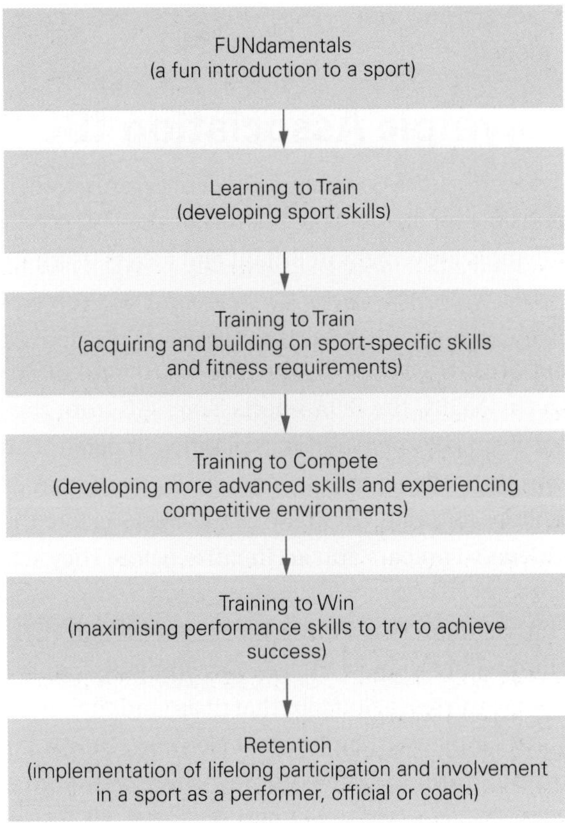

Figure 12.3 LTAD pathways

Increased participation

NGBs have been increasingly required to open up their sport to all sections of society, including those at grass-roots participation levels. This can be seen as widening the base of the sports development continuum. Ways in which an NGB can achieve sports equity include:

- developing policies linking to specific target groups, such as disabled athletes or ethnic minority athletes
- training more sport-specific coaches to encourage participation in a given sport
- developing mini-games and modified versions of the sport to encourage participation at all levels of ability, such as high-5 netball and short tennis
- making facilities more accessible, affordable and attractive to participate in, such as targeting funds at grass-roots levels and inner-city schemes
- improving awareness of the sport through publicity, advertising and use of positive role models

Tasks to tackle 12.5

How do national governing bodies of sport support and develop performers at elite performance levels?

The British Olympic Association (BOA)

The British Olympic Association (BOA) is an independent organisation, free from government control, which is responsible for all Olympic matters in the UK. It promotes interest in the Olympic Games and Olympic Movement in Britain and fosters its ideals.

Leading Team GB

The BOA provides support for Team GB in the lead up to, and duration of, the Olympic Games. Working with the NGBs, the BOA selects Team GB from the best sportsmen and women. Every aspect of Team GB's preparation is planned in detail. This involves organising visits to the host city prior to the Olympic Games and creating an exclusive preparation camp with the best facilities for Team GB to use in the weeks before the Games. Such measures help Team GB athletes to prepare and acclimatise before they settle into the Olympic Village.

The BOA also runs programmes that assist athletes throughout their training, not just in the lead-up to an Olympic Games. These include providing discounts at national and local sports centres, and helping athletes to find jobs that fit around their training and competition through the Olympic and Paralympic Employment Network (OPEN).

Funding is gained through appeals and corporate sponsorship, to enable performers to compete at the Olympics. The money is used to pay for travel, kit and attendance at preparation camps such as the Olympic Training Centre.

Olympic Medical Institute

Team GB athletes have access to the best medical advice and support whenever they need it at the Olympic Medical Institute (OMI). A team of highly experienced doctors, nutritionists, physiotherapists and other medical personnel ensure that athletes recover quicker from injury and are in top condition to compete at the Olympic Games.

The Youth Olympic Festivals

These give young Team GB athletes the opportunity to compete at a multi-sport event and get a taste of the Olympic experience. In association with the Olympic governing bodies, the BOA selects and manages a team for the Youth Festivals.

The British Olympic Foundation

As the charitable arm of the BOA, the British Olympic Foundation (BOF) is committed to inspiring through sport and education. The BOF aims to raise the profile and understanding of the Olympic principles and ideals through a wide range of activities. The BOF also aims to encourage participation in sport and hosts many events that promote physical activity and the benefits of leading a healthy lifestyle.

The BOA and London 2012

One of the key aims of the BOA is to coordinate bids to host the Olympics, culminating in securing the 2012 event. For London 2012, the BOA aims to field the largest and most competitive Team GB ever, with the ambition to finish fourth in the overall medal table. This goal was set before the team's Beijing Olympic success, which saw the target achieved 4 years early.

There are four organisations responsible for delivering the 2012 Olympic Games. Known as key stakeholders, they are the BOA, the UK Government, the Mayor of London, and the London Organising Committee of the Olympic Games (LOCOG). Each organisation has specific commitments that it must fulfil and its own dedicated role in the project.

The BOA's role is defined by three commitments:

- to secure success in the Olympic Games
- to promote, through sport, the Olympic ideals across the 2012 programme
- to deliver a viable London Olympic Institute

Sports Coach UK

This is the only organisation in the UK dedicated to providing an infrastructure geared towards better coaches. It is a charitable organisation funded by UK Sport and Sport England. It also earns its own income by selling its products through Coachwise Limited (Sports Coach UK's wholly owned trading company). Sports Coach UK operates at the level of policy, NGBs and individual coaches.

Sports Coach UK aims to develop more professional coaching policies and set higher national standards of coaching. It already organises and maintains the Coaching for Teachers scheme, designed to improve standards of coaching in schools, the UK Coaching Certificate and the World Class Coaching system. It works with, and supports, NGBs in developing skilled coaches through its resources and courses. Assistance is also offered to NGBs via a network of Coaching Development Officers in England to offer 'coaching support', for example in designing coaching plans and setting performance objectives.

For individual coaches, Sports Coach UK offers workshops, as well as resources such as coaching DVDs, covering a wide range of subjects and applicable to all levels of coaching, including high performance. It also runs the annual National Coaching Awards.

Funding of elite amateur sports performers in the UK

The National Lottery is the primary source of sports funding for elite sports performers in the UK. It provides elite individuals with funds directly via NGBs, UK Sport and the World Class Performance Programme. It also provides funds to build the high-quality facilities that elite athletes require for training and competition. The Manchester Velodrome, for example, has received large injections of Lottery funding since it was built in 1994. The venue has been the home of the hugely successful British cycling team and saw nine gold medals for British cyclists in the World Championships staged there in March 2008.

Lottery funding also goes to the UKSI national centres so that appropriate support services and scientific analysis can aid the development of elite performers. At a grass roots level, Lottery funding maintains the NGBs' Whole Sport Plans to develop sports from the foundation through to elite levels.

SportsAid is another important source of funding to the amateur elite sports performer. It is a self-financing organisation, which gets its money from individual donations, charities, private sponsors and fund-raising events.

SportsAid has a number of criteria that it uses to allocate funding to individuals. It specifically supports:

- young, up-and-coming performers in education
- those with 'potential'/NGB recommendation
- those with a proven financial need (i.e. on a low income)
- those not supported by other sources, such as Lottery funds

Top tip

SportsAid's charitable status gives it tax benefits and encourages donations.

Top tip

SportsAid funds performers with disabilities and of any age.

Practice makes perfect

1 Identify key characteristics of World Games events such as the Olympics. *(2 marks)*

2 Outline the role of national institutes of sport in the development of elite performers in the home countries. *(4 marks)*

3 Outline ways in which Sports Coach UK is having an impact on the progression of sports performers in the UK. *(3 marks)*

4 How does the National Lottery help develop sports excellence in the UK? *(3 marks)*

5 What criteria must performers meet to receive SportsAid funding? *(2 marks)*

Chapter 13 Evaluating contemporary influences

The origins of modern-day sport and associated sporting ethics

What you need to know

By the end of this section you should be able to:

- understand and explain the social and cultural factors that have influenced the development of rational recreation from pre-industrial times to the present
- understand and explain key influences in the development of rational recreation
- understand and explain how rational recreation spread within British society, as well as globally
- explain how amateurs and professionals were viewed historically in sport compared with the present day
- define the 'contract to compete' and say how relevant it is to modern-day elite sport
- define, with appropriate examples, the concepts of gamesmanship, sportsmanship and the Olympic ideal

The development of rational recreation

The main purpose of this section of historical study is to help you understand how and why sport changed, becoming more **rational** in the post-industrial era. This will help you in comparing such developments with what had gone before, as **popular recreation** in the pre-industrial period.

Key terms

Rational recreation: the post-industrial development of sport which was characterised by respectability, regularity, stringent administration and codification.

Codification: the creation and maintenance of rules.

Top tip

Some of the characteristics of **r**ational **r**ecreation can be remembered with the letter 'R' (**r**ule based, **r**egular, **r**espectable, **r**egional).

Characteristics of rational recreation

As society developed following urbanisation and the Industrial Revolution, sport became more 'rational'. It was played regularly, to set rules, in purpose-built facilities. There was an ethos of fair play in an atmosphere of respectability and gambling was controlled. Elements of both amateurism and professionalism were evident as sport became rationalised.

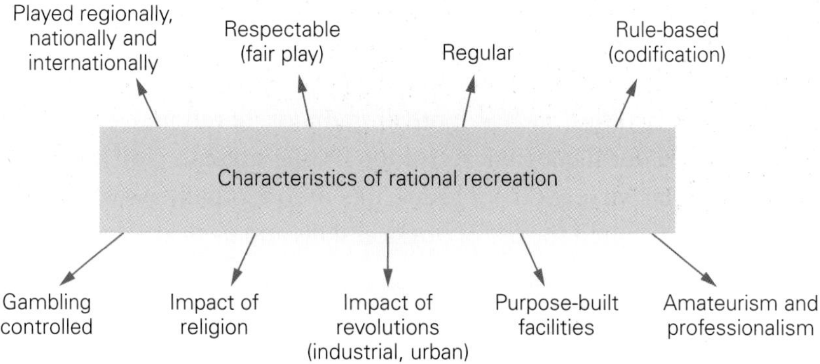

Figure 13.1 Summary of the characteristics of rational recreation

Tasks to tackle 13.1

Without reference to notes, copy and complete the following diagram, listing the characteristics of rational recreation.

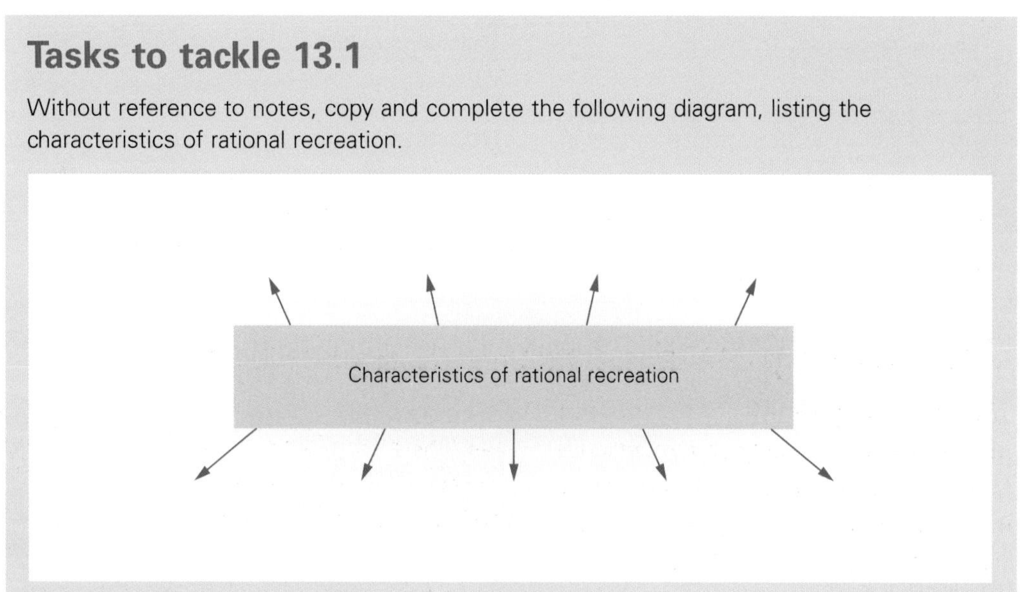

The differences between popular recreation and rational recreation were largely the result of cultural changes as society became more industrialised and organised. Rational recreation was played in urban areas to codified rules, whereas rurally played popular recreation only had simple, unwritten rules. While rational recreation was respectable, with gambling controlled, popular recreation often involved

Rational recreation	Popular recreation
Regular competitions, regionally, nationally and internationally	Occasional events/competitions held locally
Strict codification	Simple, unwritten rules
Respectable, fair play, non-violent	Violent, unruly, cruel
Control of gambling	Wagering
Purpose-built facilities	Natural/simple environment
Urban	Rural
Skill based/tactical	Strength based/few tactics

Table 13.1 A comparison of rational recreation characteristics with those of popular recreation

cruelty, violence and wagering. Regular regional, national and international competitions in rational recreation were in contrast to the irregular, local events during the popular recreation era.

The purpose-built facilities, such as football stadiums, of rational recreation replaced the natural resources used during popular recreation. While strength (and often brute force) was important for popular recreation activities, like mob football, association football as its rational counterpart required the use of physical skills and tactical awareness.

Tasks to tackle 13.2

Copy and complete the following table, which summarises key differences between popular recreation in pre-industrial Britain and rational recreation in post-industrial Britain.

Popular recreation	Rational recreation
(1) Local	(1)
(2)	(2) Codified
(3)	(3) Respectable
(4) Occasional	(4)
(5) Rural	(5)
(6) Natural resources	(6)

Social and cultural influences on rational recreation

Rational recreation differed from popular recreation in relation to who was playing, and where, when and how it was being played. Such changes reflected societal and cultural change. By the mid-nineteenth century, Britain was an **urbanised** society and fully industrialised.

The early stages of the **Industrial Revolution** had many negative impacts on the working classes.

Key terms

Urbanisation: a massive expansion in the number of people living in towns and cities as a result of industrialisation.

Industrial Revolution: deemed to cover the century 1750–1850, this period marked a change in Britain from a feudal, rural society into an industrialised, capitalist society controlled by a powerful urban middle class.

Top tip

In exam questions, it is important that you can compare the characteristics of rational recreation with popular recreation and explain the socio-cultural factors implementing such changes.

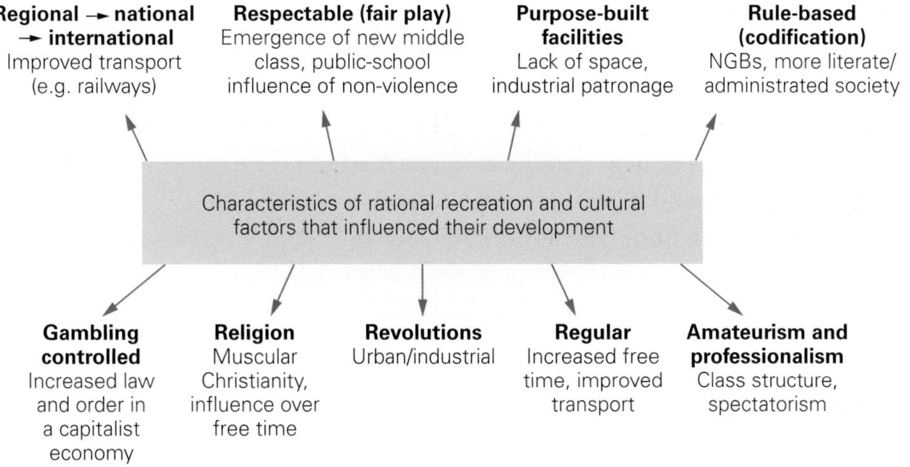

Figure 13.2 Social and cultural influences on the characteristics of rational recreation

Urbanisation on a massive scale saw the lower classes migrating into newly formed cities, with a consequent loss of space. Overcrowding was often accompanied by poor living and working conditions, as labour shifted from the seasonal work of agriculture to the 'machine time' of factories — often involving 12-hour shifts. Coupled with low incomes, workers' health was often poor and there was little energy or time left to play sports. Furthermore, the workers' traditional sports — so-called mob games and blood sports such as cock fighting and bare knuckle boxing — were criminalised, leading to the loss of the right to play.

In the second half of the nineteenth century, conditions improved and played a key role in developing sport in a more rational manner. Hygiene was improved in the workplace and at home, with a subsequent improvement in workers' health. Several laws, the Factory Acts, gave workers more time off, such as a half day on Saturdays. Together with the huge improvements in transport and communications, this led to a rise in **spectatorism** — for example, watching football. The Football Association was founded in 1863 and heralded as 'the People's Game'.

Using the railways, both spectators and players could now travel further and faster, giving increased time in which to play and an ability to follow a team. Following a local team encouraged a sense of identity that benefited the workers and their employers. In reality, the costs involved were still large and workers were often reliant on the benevolence of their employers for special trips. Entire trains were sometimes hired for these occasions, which could either involve sport or a trip to a seaside town. The railways did, however, influence the establishment of national leagues.

Top tip

It is important to be aware that the emergence of sport for the working class masses was hard won. Initially, migration to towns was met with gloom, ill health and poverty for many. It was only in the second half of the nineteenth century that things began to improve for the working classes in society in general, as well as in a sporting context.

> **Top tip**
> Sport developed rapidly in the late nineteenth century. Advancements in transport played a role in enabling such developments to occur.

Regular fixtures grew up between towns with stations, with matches being played regularly on a regional and national basis. This increased the need for a standardised set of rules.

The development of a new middle class changed ways of playing sport, and it became more acceptable. Those with a public school education had a strong affection for the sports ethos they had learned at school. They took their various school versions of games with them to university, particularly Oxford and Cambridge. The bringing together of these 'games that were a bit like football' and the agreeing of a set of standard rules is known as the 'melting pot'. Cambridge Rules Football, for example, was widely played in the 1840s. Note that the development of a common set of rules and the creation of NGBs by the upper and middle classes coincided with the need for such measures by the increasingly sporting and literate working classes. The control and running of sporting clubs was seen as a business opportunity by some middle-class entrepreneurs.

> **Key term**
> **Industrial patronage:** factory teams, including Arsenal and Manchester United, were set up as a way of reducing absenteeism in the factory workforce.

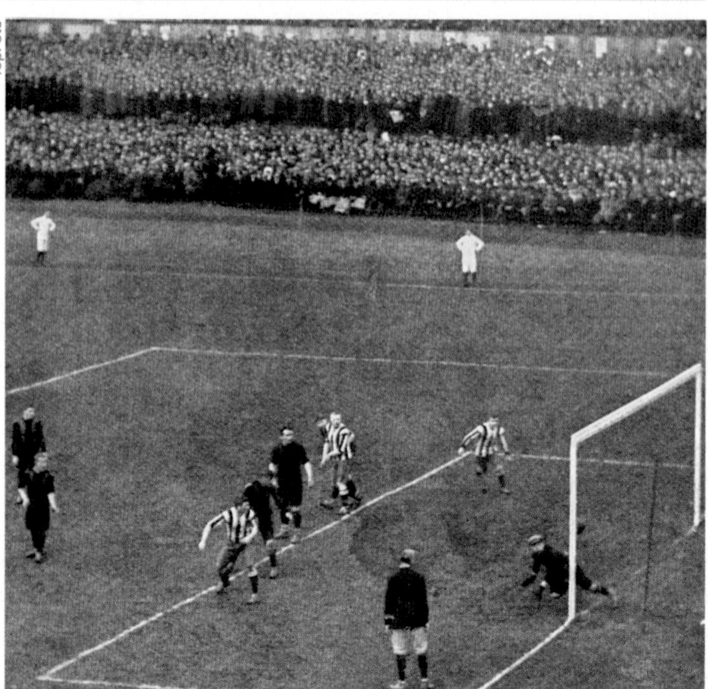
TopFoto

Newcastle scores its only goal in a 3–1 defeat by Wolverhampton Wanderers in May 1908

Former public school boys grew up to gain prominence — and therefore power — in industrial and religious circles (see pages 142–43). The money and patronage that came with the middle class improved provision for recreation and sport. Factory owners set up factory teams, provided paid holidays and paid for new, purpose-built facilities. Interestingly, it was the lack of space in the urban environment that led to the reduction in size of the playing area, or pitch. Earlier versions of football moved freely over rural spaces. The crowding of the urban environment was also a contributing factor in the rise of spectatorism, as there were large numbers of people looking for entertainment.

'Soccer' was played both as an amateur game for gentlemen as well as a professional game for 'the people' (i.e. the working class).

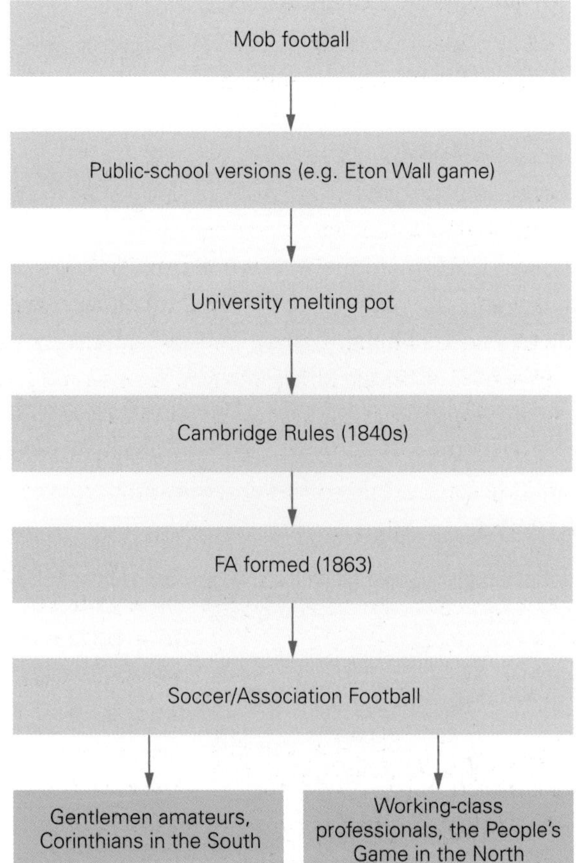

Figure 13.3 The emergence of association football from mob football

Ex-public school boys formed the Football Association in 1863. However, massive crowds and increased demand for regular matches led to professionalism being made legal in 1885 and the establishment of the Football League in 1888. The Rugby Football Union was established in 1871. This ended the practice of playing half a game of soccer and the other half of rugby in order to meet the tastes of all concerned!

As the game became formalised, clearly defined playing rules and official roles (such as referees) emerged. Violence was controlled by the laws of the game and spectating became more organised, for example with the introduction of stands at grounds.

The public school values of athleticism and fair play soon spread to the lower classes (particularly as they were written into the rules of the only allowable sports) and football became a good job to aspire to. Professional football was seen as a chance to escape urban deprivation and bad working conditions. **Broken time payments** further encouraged the participation of players and spectators who could not otherwise afford to miss work.

Key term

Broken time payments: finance/money paid to the working classes for time they had to take off to play sport.

Table 13.2 Summary of the working conditions affecting sports participation in the late nineteenth century

Industrialisation	Factory machines required long working shifts as they had to be kept running in order to make a profit
Holiday patterns	These were regularised for all workers — a single week or day (initially without pay)
Free time	The little free time available was organised to discourage absenteeism from work; Church attendance on Sundays was 'encouraged', so Sunday sports time was limited
Working hours	Gradual decrease from 72 hours a week; various Factory Acts led to the adoption of Saturday half day/early closing day for shops, which meant more free time to watch and play sport
Urbanisation	A lack of space required purpose-built facilities; gradual increase in public provision of parks and baths; spectatorism at football
Patronage (of urban middle classes)	Excursions were paid for by some bosses; workers' sports teams developed and purpose-built facilities were provided

Tasks to tackle 13.3

(a) How did the 'half day' Factory Acts facilitate the development of sport at the end of the nineteenth century?

(b) List and explain four social/cultural factors that influenced the development of rationalised sports and pastimes in late nineteenth-century Britain.

The influence of the Church

During the nineteenth century, football became increasingly popular in public schools. Initially there was no clear differentiation between football and rugby as the rules had not been formally established.

The educational reformer Dr Thomas Arnold encouraged games at Rugby School and viewed them as a useful way of controlling the surplus energy of the scholars. His ideas were based on Christian principles linked to the cult of athleticism to provide the boys with a sense of discipline, moral fibre and responsibility, and it was such ideals that saw the development and expansion of the British empire. (Missionaries introduced rugby to the Maoris in New Zealand and the Indian FA was established with the help of an English international soccer player who was a priest.)

The popularity of games in this era was also enhanced by the writings of the Rev. Charles Kingsley who promoted the development of a 'healthy mind and body' and whose morality was encapsulated in I Corinthians 6:19, advocating that the body should be a temple of the Lord. Such was the philosophy of the Muscular Christians, who used games like football and rugby to promote Christianity among poorer sections of the community. Organised games or rational recreation were viewed as countering the vices that were reported in towns and cities. The Church could now associate itself with sport as it was far more rational and respectable than its previous 'popular recreation' counterpart.

Today, professional clubs that originated from church teams organised by the clergy include Aston Villa, Birmingham City, Bolton Wanderers, Burnley, Fulham, Liverpool, Queens Park Rangers, Southampton, Swindon and Wolverhampton Wanderers. There were also Church connections with northern rugby clubs. For example, Salford was formed in 1873 as Cavendish FC by members of Cavendish Street Chapel Sunday School and Runcorn was formed in 1876 as a section of the Runcorn Young Men's Christian FA Athletic Club.

The Rev. Frank Marshall was a leading crusader of amateur rugby (and highly critical of professionalism), who wrote *Football: The Rugby Union Game,* published in 1892. When rugby league became professional in 1895, increasing violence and drunkenness among players and spectators led to the loss of Church support.

Throughout the twentieth century, the influence of the clergy on sport was still apparent and well documented. The Bishop of Liverpool (1975–97), the Rt Rev. David Sheppard, played cricket for Cambridge and Sussex and captained England in 1954.

Puritan-style Sabbatarianism (strict adherence to resting — including no sport — on the Sabbath) did not disappear. The box-office success *Chariots of Fire* featured the life of Eric Liddell who was a missionary in China and competed in the 440 yards in the 1926 Paris Olympics, winning gold. He refused to race on a Sunday. Triple jump world record holder and Olympic gold medallist in Sydney 2000, Jonathan Edwards, also refused to compete on a Sunday on religious grounds.

Monarchs, aristocrats, industrialists, businessmen, professionals and, in the late-Victorian era, artisans, tradesmen, shopkeepers and the industrial proletariat have all had an impact on the growth of games. However, the Victorian clergy, through their involvement in sport, were able to communicate with the population on a daily basis through the common denominator of a popularly held interest and so relay their faith to the working classes in the towns and cities of nineteenth-century England.

The formation of national governing bodies of sport

Many national governing bodies (NGBs) for sport in England were formed during the late 1800s. As described above, the ex-public schoolboys who formed them were influenced by a number of factors, including the need for codification to ensure that sports were played in a more uniform manner. With more fixtures and leisure clubs being formed, teams required not only rules but also competitions and leagues to play in. In addition, the development of professionalism and commercialism in sport in the late 1800s needed 'controlling', as the middle classes wanted to maintain control of sport and preserve their amateur ideals.

Top tip

The influence of ex-public schoolboys who went on to universities and led the formation of many NGBs is of key importance.

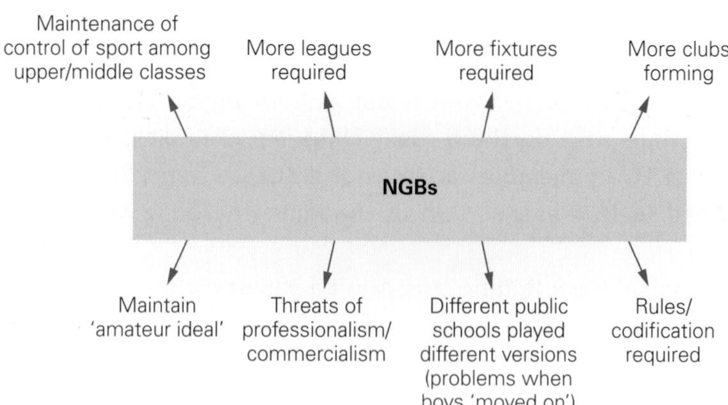

Figure 13.4 Factors affecting the formation of NGBs

Rationalisation of sport: case studies

Bathing/swimming

A number of 'spa towns', such as Bath and Malvern, developed historically for the amusement of the upper classes. Wealthy individuals paid to drink or immerse themselves in the local water as a cure for ill-health. A number of 'river towns' developed later and organised swimming and competitive swimming as a therapeutic activity, for example in London. 'Seaside towns' also emerged, with a belief in the therapeutic effects of immersion in water. By the late nineteenth century, improvements in the rail network meant that the working classes could

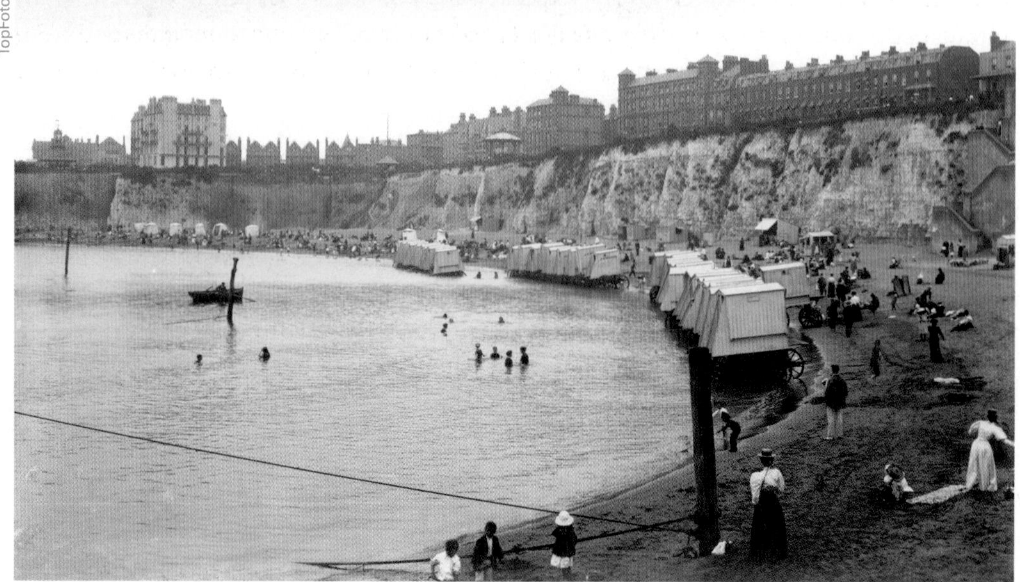

Seaside towns became popular during Victorian times. The bathing machines on the right of the photograph were wheeled into the sea, allowing bathers to change inside them and to bathe in privacy.

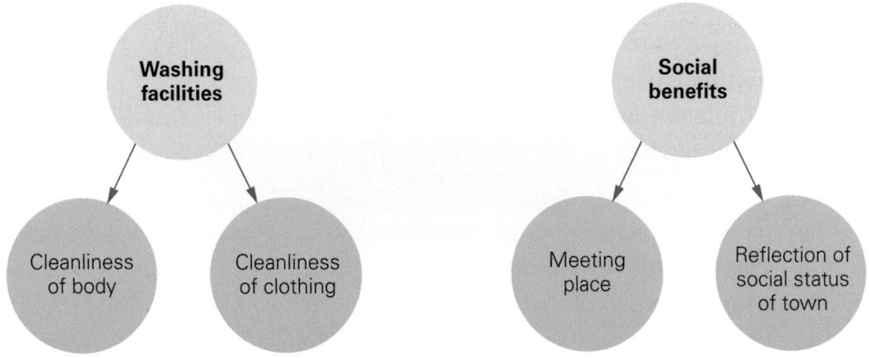

Figure 13.5 Functions of public baths in the second half of the nineteenth century

more easily visit seaside towns, such as Blackpool, from northern industrial towns, and gain access to these activities.

> **Key term**
>
> **Spa movement:** part of the Regency fashion, around 1800, for the upper classes to stay at elite watering places, or 'baths', where they took the 'water cure'.

The Wash House Acts (1846–48) led to money being given to towns to build 'public baths'. The primary aim was to clean up the working classes, promote exercise and combat the spread of diseases such as cholera (and ultimately to increase efficiency at work). Disease had become more widespread as a result of urban pollution of rivers. The working classes paid a small fee to visit the 'second-class facility' in the public baths. The middle classes used the 'first-class facility', consisting of Turkish baths and plunge pools, which facilitated competitive races. Amateur clubs and NGBs were formed as swimming became a 'respectable' activity, with the Amateur Swimming Association (ASA) emerging in 1884.

Athletics

Prior to industrialisation, rural fairs were popular gatherings and often included running and throwing competitions as demonstrations of speed and strength. Running contests of various kinds were extremely popular. In the eighteenth century, for example, pedestrianism (a sort of long-distance walking race) involved large cash prizes and extensive gambling. Exploitation by the gentry was common, however, with footmen being raced against each other for the gain of their masters.

As England became increasingly urbanised, rural fairs were exchanged for urban festivals, taking the sports to a wider, more organised, arena. Urban festivals took place in most large towns and cities in the early nineteenth century, attracting huge crowds (spectatorism) and widespread wagering.

However, the wagering on races encouraged cheating, such as race fixing, which was frowned upon by the middle classes and there was a desire to maintain separation from such negative aspects of athletics. By 1850, most major cities had purpose-built tracks, which allowed more stringent timekeeping and the beginning of record keeping, all of which meant increased organisation and rationalisation of the sport.

The Amateur Athletic Club (AAC) was formed in 1866 as an exclusive amateur club. Its organisers wanted to dissociate respectable Modern Athletics from the corrupted professional form and they adopted an exclusion clause — essentially banning labourers (working men) from athletics. This form of athletics was illustrated by the first Oxford–Cambridge Varsity meeting in 1864 and saw the start of sports days being embedded in the public school system.

The AAC was the forerunner of the Amateur Athletic Association, which emerged in 1880. The definition employed by this body was that 'an amateur is one who has never competed for a money prize or a staked bet, or who has never taught, pursued, or assisted in the practice of athletic exercises as a means of obtaining a livelihood'.

Athletics is now 'open' as a sport, with professionals competing on the world circuit for prize and appearance money. But amateur athletics still exists at club level for many.

Tasks to tackle 13.4

Describe the emergence of 'amateur athletics' during the late nineteenth century.

Amateurism and professionalism

There have been differences over time in how **amateurs** and **professionals** have been viewed when involved in sports participation.

Key terms

Amateurs: not paid for sporting involvement and tend to play for the love of it.

Professionals: receive payments for sporting involvement via wagers and prize money, with extrinsic rewards an important motivator for participation.

Amateurism: This evolved in nineteenth-century Britain and involved sports participation for the love of it. Fair play and sportsmanship were more important than winning. Abiding by the spirit as well as the rules of the game were key qualities of the gentleman amateur.

In the eighteenth and nineteenth century, the 'gentleman amateur' was very wealthy and had plenty of free time in which to play sport. Sporting amateurs came from the highest social class group; they were highly respected members of society, with a public-school background. Participation in sport was viewed as a character-building exercise and 'training' was frowned upon as this would have constituted professionalism.

The middle classes who emerged as a result of the Industrial Revolution could not afford to take time off work, but at the same time they did not want to get paid to play. They admired the high cultural values of the upper-class gentleman amateur and played sport in their free time according to similar principles of **amateurism**. The middle and upper classes used the 'amateur

Table 13.3 The main differences between amateurism and professionalism

Amateurism	Professionalism
Came with the onset of the Victorian era (mid-nineteenth century onwards)	Slowly developed, with full onset coinciding with the commercialism/ media coverage of sport in the late twentieth century onwards
High morality, sportsmanship and 'gentlemanly' behaviour	Foul play, gamesmanship and cheating to gain an advantage
Games not taken too seriously; winning not important for upper classes	Win at all costs, high rewards at stake, pressure to succeed and to maintain lifestyle

code' in most sports to effectively exclude the working classes, as financially and socially this group could not meet the demands placed upon them.

The working classes were the poorest members of society and therefore had to make money from sport, otherwise they could not afford to play. The working-class professional came from a poor background and was perceived to be corruptible as he was controlled by money. He would, for example, take a bribe to throw a fight or lose a game on purpose. He was paid — by a patron or as a result of gambling — according to results; hence training was specialised and winning became the most important thing.

The status of amateurs and professionals in the late nineteenth century varied between sports. Amateur and professional cricketers could play against each other in 'gentlemen vs players' matches. Gentlemen were the amateurs and working-class players were the professionals. Rowing was originally a sport open to amateurs and professionals alike, but the gentleman amateurs disliked being beaten by social inferiors. This led to a strict amateur definition, which excluded anyone who was a 'mechanic or labourer'. This definition was abolished in 1890.

Tasks to tackle 13.5

(a) Give reasons for amateurs having higher social status than professionals in nineteenth century Britain.

(b) Explain the effects of social class for an elite level performer in Britain in the early 1900s.

Rugby football was developed at Rugby School. The game was so popular that workers in northern industrial towns adopted it, but needed to be paid to play or at least receive broken time payments. The rugby authorities (who believed in the amateur code) did not like this and it eventually led to a split in rugby: rugby union was played by amateurs from the south of the country while rugby league was played by professionals from the working classes, who had to miss work to play sport.

Ultimately, however, in the modern day, sports need to be able to survive commercially. Money enables NGBs to promote the game and also finances coaching, competitions and facilities. Players who realised that they could be paid an income from rugby league were being tempted to play the professional game and in 1996, the union game turned professional.

Table 13.4 Differences between early twentieth-century amateurs and modern-day amateurs

Early twentieth-century amateurs	Modern-day amateurs
Had a high status in sport and society	Tend to be of lower status (professionals now are of higher status)
Were the best players in their sport	Are outclassed by professionals in their sport
Were either middle or upper class and belonged to the group that controlled sport, excluding working classes (e.g. financially) from amateur sports	Blurring of amateur/professional distinctions, with less likelihood of exclusions as society is more egalitarian
Were more able to be top level performers than those of lower class	Performance at the highest level in most sports is now more open to all
Had sufficient income and leisure time to play sport for the love of it, receiving no payment	Some amateurs receive finance to pay for training, travel and living expenses (e.g. scholarships/sponsorships)

In modern-day sport, amateurs and professionals are viewed somewhat differently.

Many factors have been responsible for transforming the status of professional performers between the early twentieth century and the present day:

- All classes can now compete, so social class is no longer a barrier to participation.
- People are now respected for their talents and efforts in reaching the top, and not for their class status.
- There are high rewards for professionals, through the media and sponsorship.
- Professionals have more time to train, resulting in higher standards of performance.
- More media coverage and celebrity status for top performers act as motivators to achieve in professional sport.

The contract to compete

In all sporting situations, from a football match to a 100 m sprint, there is an unwritten contract — a mutual agreement between opponents to strive 100% to assert themselves over one another *within the rules*, allowing a *fair opportunity* to achieve the ultimate objective of winning. This contract to compete involves acceptance of the need for codes of behaviour (i.e. sportsmanship) as opposed to 'win at all costs' attitudes that lead to temptations to break rules, take drugs and other deviant behaviours.

Tasks to tackle 13.6

Why might violence by sports performers be considered as outside the 'contract to compete'?

Modern-day elite sport favours a Lombardian ethic. This 'win at all costs' attitude is named after Vince Lombardi, an American football coach during the 1960s who was famous for his motivational skills. He is credited with having said: 'Winning isn't everything; it's the only thing.' As the rewards for success become ever greater, the contract to compete is often broken.

The Olympic ideal

The idea of the contract to compete links to a view developed by Baron Pierre de Coubertin as he travelled around the English public schools. His concept views 'balance in mind and body' as highly important, with individuals encouraged to strive to do their best but at the same time to maintain respect for ethical principles. This ideal was fundamental to the modern Olympic Games when they began in 1896, founded by de Coubertin. It appears on the scoreboard at every Olympics as:

> The most important thing in the Olympic Games is not to win but to take part.

The Olympic ideal therefore involves:

- an emphasis on participation
- respect for fellow competitors
- winning as a result of one's own efforts
- improved tolerance and understanding across national boundaries

Sportsmanship

Part of the amateur code and Olympic ideal involves a 'spirit of fair play', of competing within the written or unwritten rules of a sport. This is known as **sportsmanship**.

Certain sports still have a reputation for sportsmanship and high levels of etiquette. In golf, for example, players concede a short putt in match play to an opponent, maintain silence while an opponent is playing a shot, and congratulate their opponents on a good shot or round.

Gamesmanship

In most modern-day professional sport, **gamesmanship** is very much in evidence.

With rewards for winning increasing all the time, sports performers have employed a number of underhand tactics that are still within the rules...just. Examples include time wasting in football, sledging (verbal antagonism), over appealing (putting pressure on the umpire to give a batsman as out) in cricket, and faking an injury time-out in tennis to disrupt an opponent's concentration.

Key term

Gamesmanship: attempting to gain an advantage in sport by stretching the rules to their limit.

Tasks to tackle 13.7

Write 'S', 'C' or 'G' as appropriate after each of the following six sports scenarios.

S = Sportsmanship C = Cheating G = Gamesmanship

(a) Taking injury time-outs in tennis

(b) Diving to win a penalty in football

(c) Conceding a putt close to the hole in golf match play

(d) Clapping when the opposing netball team scores

(e) An athlete taking drugs to improve speed/power

(f) Over appealing in cricket

Practice makes perfect

1 Explain the changes in football from the 'popular' to the 'rational' form with reference to:
(a) working conditions
(b) urbanisation
(c) transport *(6 marks)*

2 Discuss the concepts of amateurism and professionalism in association football during the second half of the nineteenth century. *(3 marks)*

3 Modern-day sport is increasingly about 'winning at all costs', with cheating and gamesmanship more evident than in the past. Explain what is meant by the term gamesmanship. *(3 marks)*

4 What are the effects of fair play on a sport or sporting situation? *(3 marks)*

Chapter 14

Evaluating contemporary influences

Sport, deviance and the law

What you need to know

By the end of this chapter, you should be able to:

- explain positive and negative forms of deviance in sport in relation to players and spectators, using examples to illustrate your answer
- list and explain the causes and implications of violence in sport and give strategies for preventing violence by both performers and spectators
- list and explain the reasons why elite performers use illegal drugs to aid performance, and discuss the implications this has for the performer and sport itself
- discuss arguments for and against drug taking and testing, and give ways in which drug taking can be discouraged or eliminated
- explain how the law is increasingly relevant to sporting performers, officials and spectators

In Chapter 13 we covered the traditional values of amateurism, sportsmanship and the Olympic ideal. These values have underpinned the British sport system and as a nation we have viewed them positively. However, as we know, the sports world is also full of behaviour that goes against these principles and ethics. This type of behaviour can be referred to as **deviant behaviour**, or **deviancy**.

Behaviour can be criminally deviant — that is, against the law — or morally deviant, whereby no law has been broken but society would generally not consider the behaviour in a positive light. In March 2008, for example, Liverpool footballer Javier Mascherano received a lot of criticism for his refusal to leave the field of play after being sent off in a game against Manchester United. At the start of the 2008/2009 football season, the FA introduced its 'Respect' campaign to try to eliminate such disrespect towards officials and improve football's image at all levels of the game.

If we consider the phrase 'against society's norms and values', it is clear that someone or some group in society has imposed their set of ideas on others. This group would be considered the dominant group in society and in the UK this dominance could be deemed to be white, male and middle class. This is the group that has the most control and power in terms of distribution of resources and decision making at the highest levels. Therefore, groups of people who fall outside

Key terms

Deviancy: behaviour that goes against society's general norms and values.

Negative deviancy: behaviour that goes against the normal values of society to the detriment of the rules or the player's health.

Positive deviancy: an over-adherence to the rules that govern society, often to the detriment of the player's health.

these boundaries may well hold opposing views and opinions and have different behaviour patterns, but this would not necessarily mean they were 'wrong'. Thus deviancy is relative and deviants may be the victims of a power system that makes the rules.

Sports performers become part of a community bonded by a sense of commitment and are often encouraged to behave in ways that would not be accepted in other areas of life. 'On the field', deviant behaviour can be caused by the pressure of the media, coaches, sponsorship deals and so on. If the athlete's behaviour breaks the rules of the sport, this can be dealt with appropriately. However, a culture may develop that accepts this type of behaviour and even deems it necessary for the sake of winning (for example, diving to win a penalty in football).

> **Top tip**
>
> Questions on negative deviancy — for example, aggression, violence, doping and hooliganism — are popular in the AQA exam. However, make sure you understand positive deviancy as well.

There are two types of deviancy you need to be aware of:

- **Negative deviancy** in sporting situations can include violations such as deliberately fouling another player or taking performance-enhancing drugs. The main motivation is to 'win at all costs', i.e. Lombardianism (see page 148).
- **Positive deviancy** involves athletes behaving in ways that would be acceptable in other spheres of life, but taking that behaviour to extremes. This can be classed as over-conformity to the sporting ethic. An example of positive deviancy is where an athlete is encouraged to over-train or perform when injured; in other aspects of life we would not encourage someone to cause further damage to his or her health. The motivation for positive deviancy may include not letting people down rather than simply wanting to be the best.

The next part of this chapter focuses on the causes and implications of negative deviancy, and possible means of combating deviant behaviour.

Violence among sports performers

All sport involves some sort of **conflict**, which can be positive or negative. This is the essence of competition. If it is controlled, conflict is functional, but uncontrolled conflict can soon become dysfunctional — that is, negative to the players, officials, spectators and sport itself.

We attempt to control any conflict situations by channelling the **aggression** in a positive way, which can act as a catharsis or stress relief. Channelled aggression or **balanced tension** is the ability to utilise all your resources to achieve optimum performance without using unlawful or unethical strategies.

> **Key terms**
>
> **Conflict:** change and/or progress is made by one group at the expense of another.
>
> **Aggression:** the intention to harm another human being either verbally or mentally.
>
> **Balanced tension:** a degree of stress that is productive because it is controlled and channelled.

Conflict appears in many forms among sports performers:

- At an individual level this may be due to emotional intensity. For example, when striving to achieve a personal best, or when a match is charged (such as a local Derby), the performer may be overly psyched up and unable to cope with any subsequent failure.
- Conflict can develop within a team, for example between top goal scorers.
- Conflict may exist against another team, for example for historical reasons. There may also be provocation by the opposition, for example verbal sledging.
- Spectators can impact on players' stress levels and players have been known to become aggressive or abusive towards a crowd. Eric Cantona, for example, struck out against a

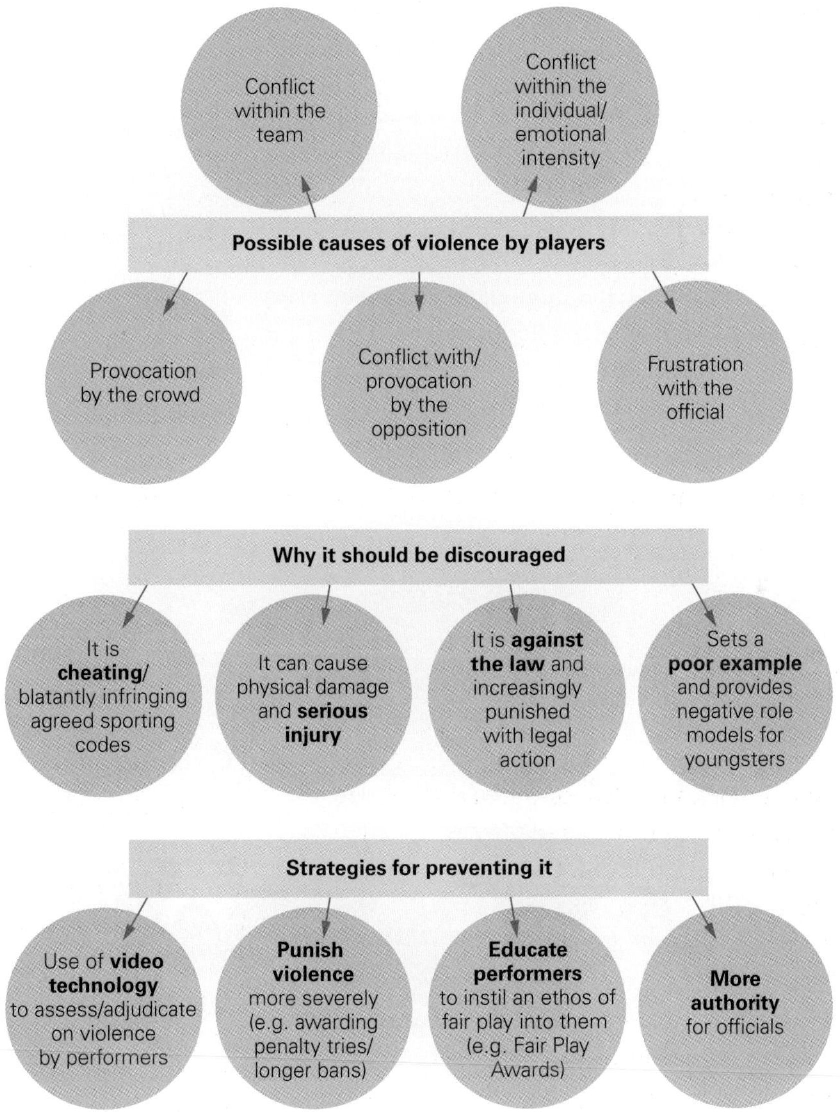

Figure 14.1 Summary of the causes and effects of violence by players

spectator after being sent off while playing for Manchester United in 1995. He claimed the spectator was racially abusive and threw a missile, but his response (a kung-fu-style kick to the face) resulted in a community sentence.
- Conflict frequently arises with officials, for example when disagreeing with decisions made.

Conflict can also be determined by the nature of the activity, for example contact or non-contact sports.

Violence among spectators: football hooliganism

> **Key term**
> **Hooligan:** a disorderly, violent person commonly associated with the game of football.

Spectators are not able to release their tension in the same way as the performers who are actively exerting themselves. This can cause frustration, which can lead to violence.

Professional football is by far the most popular spectator sport in Britain. Today it is estimated that around 4–5 million people attend football matches in England and Wales every year. However, this number is smaller than it used to be and there are many complex reasons for this, such as changing leisure patterns — many individuals prefer to shop rather than watch a football match. However, many people blame football's relative decline up until the mid-1980s on football hooliganism.

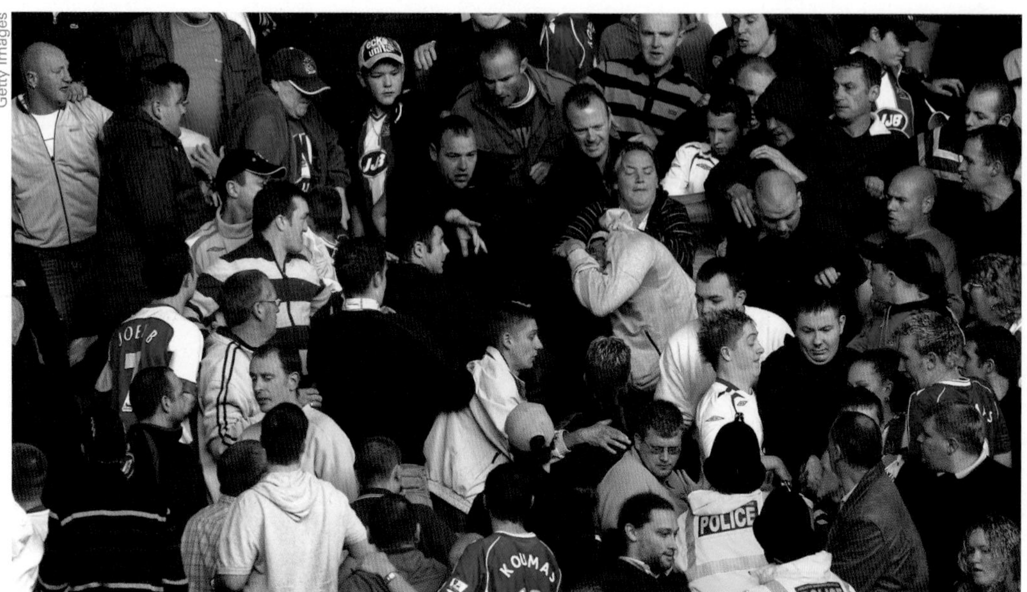

Getty Images

Crowd violence during the Wigan versus Liverpool Premier League game in September 2007

Although football hooliganism was not recognised by the government and the media as a serious problem until the 1960s, hooligan behaviour at football matches, particularly in England, has a long history. 'Roughs' were regularly reported as causing trouble at matches in the professional game's early years at the end of the nineteenth century, on occasions attacking and stoning referees as well as the visiting players. It was not until the early 1960s, however, that media coverage of football began to report hooliganism at matches regularly. It was around this time that football hooliganism in England began to take on a more cohesive and organised appearance.

Theories of hooliganism

Most of the evidence on hooliganism offenders suggests that they are in their late teens or early 20s (though some 'leaders' are older). They are mainly in manual or lower clerical occupations or, to a lesser extent, unemployed and they come mainly from working-class backgrounds. This is not always the case, however. Perhaps unsurprisingly, London hooligans tend to be more affluent than their counterparts elsewhere. Sometimes spontaneous and 'random' in their acts of violence, hooligans can also be involved in political conspiracies and the more formal organisation of hooligan assaults.

Table 14.1 Football hooliganism – some general theories and how valid they are

General theories	Arguments against
Young working-class males releasing aggression, thrill seeking, fuelled by alcohol	Lack of evidence that working-class males are any more or any less aggressive than other males
Nationalism (seeing other countries' fans as an enemy, as encouraged by media hype, e.g. Germany versus England)	Not all international spectators/other sports act like this
Reaction by working-class fans to the takeover of football by middle-class spectators	Hooligans come from a wide range of social backgrounds
Lack of punishment by authorities	Stricter punishments are being given out by the authorities
Violent on-pitch actions by players and poor officiating provoke off-pitch violence	Some 'violent' sports are not linked to hooliganism (e.g. rugby); on-pitch behaviour is well controlled

If football hooliganism were to re-emerge in the twenty-first century game in England, the consequences would be severe. Individual performers, and football itself, might lose sponsorship and funding since businesses seek a positive image for their products and also because audiences would move away from the sport, leading to a declining market for those products. The financial implications would also affect the media, as declining coverage would lead to commercial losses. New talent could be put off playing football due to the negative image of the sport. Fans, even non-violent ones, could face a ban from attending matches at home and abroad. Teams could face a loss of points and elimination from competitions. Ultimately, the violence could spread into wider society.

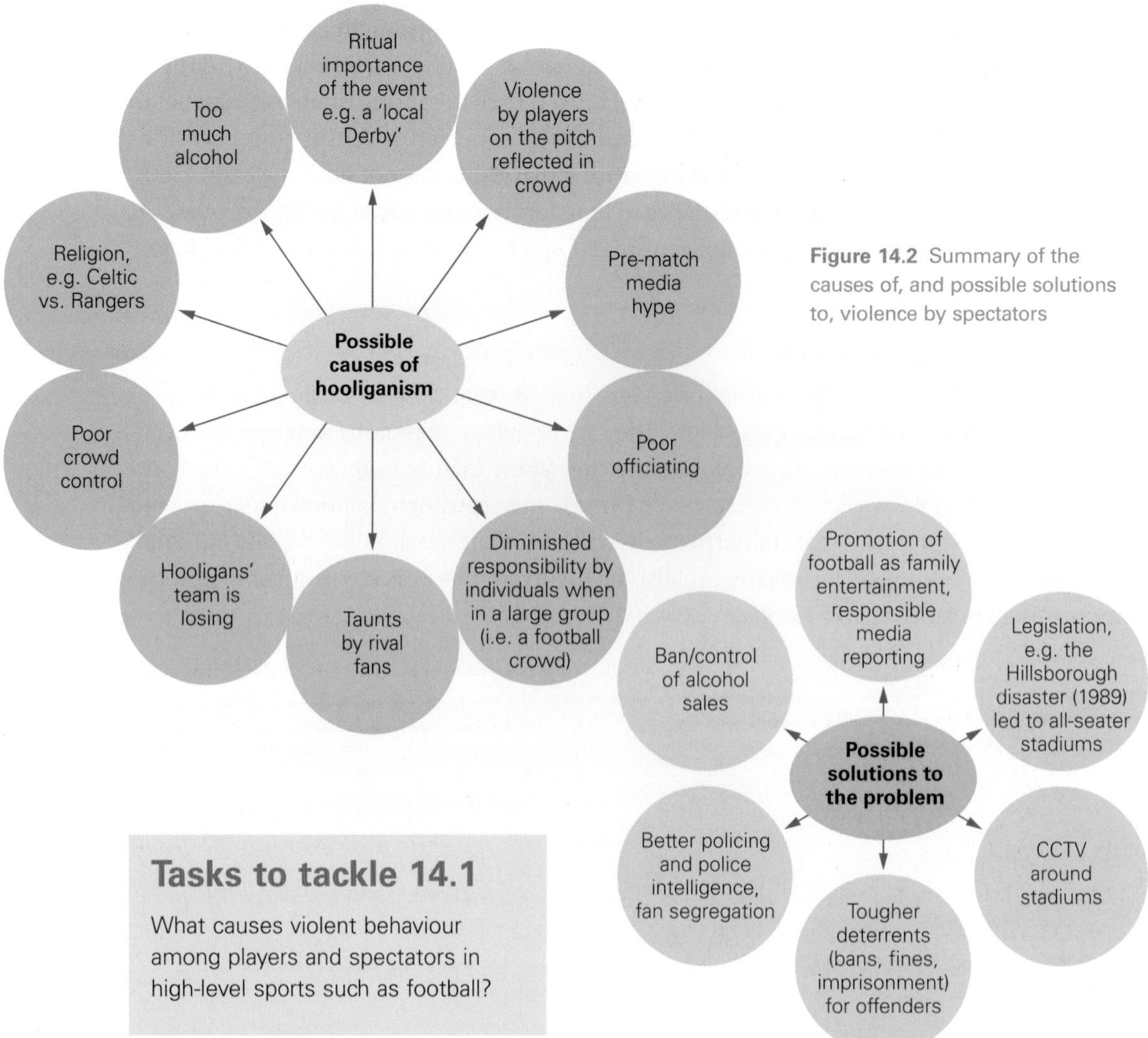

Figure 14.2 Summary of the causes of, and possible solutions to, violence by spectators

> **Tasks to tackle 14.1**
>
> What causes violent behaviour among players and spectators in high-level sports such as football?

Drug taking in sport

It is part of the Olympic oath to take part in the Games '...without doping and without drugs in the true spirit of competition'. In other words, avoiding drugs is within the contract to compete that each Olympic athlete undertakes. The desire to win at all costs in the highly competitive world of modern-day sport, however, means that performers continue to take drugs illegally despite the obvious risks attached. The AQA specification requires an understanding of the issues surrounding reasons why sports performers take drugs and ways in which drug taking can be eliminated. It is useful therefore to have an overview of the types of drugs used in the world of elite sports performance, as illustrated by Table 14.2.

Table 14.2 Examples of different drugs, why sports performers use them and their possible side effects

Type of drug	Reasons for use	Side effects	Sporting examples
Anabolic steroids (artificially produced male hormones, e.g. testosterone)	Promote muscle growth Permit harder/longer training without muscle fatigue Increased aggression	Females develop male features Liver/heart damage Mood swings/over-aggression	Power/explosive events, such as 100 m sprinting and weightlifting
Narcotics (painkillers)	Reduce pain Mask injury	Highly addictive Respiratory problems Nausea	All sports (all potentially involve injury)
Stimulants (stimulate the body both physically and mentally, e.g. caffeine/amphetamines)	Reduce tiredness/increase endurance Increase alertness	Rise in blood pressure/temperature Addiction Irregular/faster heartbeat	Cycling
Beta-blockers	Steady nerves Stop trembling	Lower heart rate and blood pressure	Sports where fine motor control is required, such as archery and snooker
Diuretics (remove body fluid)	Lose weight quickly	Dehydration Dizziness Fainting	Sports with weight requirements, such as horse racing and boxing
Naturally occurring hormones (e.g. EPO, erythropoietin)	Build and mend muscle Increase oxygen transport	Muscle wasting EPO can increase red blood cell count to dangerous levels	Distance runners Swimmers
Blood doping (removal of blood 2–3 months before competition and re-injection a week before the event to increase the number of red blood cells)	Body has more energy to work	Heart attack, stroke and pulmonary embolism	Endurance events, such as marathon running and long-distance cycling

The reasons why athletes take performance-enhancing drugs can be grouped as follows:

- **physiological reasons**, as listed in Table 14.2, such as building muscle strength (anabolic steroids), steadying nerves (beta blockers), increasing energy (EPO) and the ability to train harder
- **psychological reasons**, such as increasing aggression (anabolic steroids), raising confidence (stimulants)
- **social reasons**, such as financial reward, giving entertainment, becoming famous, and pressure to win from coaches, peers, the media, sponsors and the athletes themselves

Top tip

You are not required to have an in-depth knowledge of the psychological effects of drugs in sport, but a basic understanding of the main types used, their effects and side effects is useful background knowledge linked to the social issues surrounding their usage in sport.

Why drugs are banned from sport

Performance-enhancing drugs give an unfair and unnatural advantage to the users. This is seen as against the true nature of sporting competition. The illegality of drug taking is therefore built into the ethics, and consequently the official rules, of many sporting organisations such as the International Olympic Committee (IOC). These rules attempt to prevent drug taking by imposing consequences, such as loss of medals, shame and a ban, on drug takers. It can be argued that any perceived lack of punishment reduces the deterrent for athletes considering taking drugs.

Drug taking has associated health risks. These can be severe, leading to addiction, illness and even death. As a result, many performance-enhancing drugs are illegal. Sporting rules therefore merely reflect the laws of the land in making them illegal in the sporting arena too.

Due to its unfair and immoral nature, drug taking is associated with a negative sporting image. A sport tainted by drug taking can provide negative role models, lose its audience, and consequently lose earnings through sponsorship. The 2007 Tour de France, for example, was dubbed the Tour de Farce by the media due to the high number of competitors who failed drugs tests. A number of teams lost sponsors as a result.

Should drugs in sport be legalised?

Does banning drugs give their effects a perceived value that in reality is not as great? Does ineffective drugs testing mean that not all cheats are caught, and that others are therefore choosing to attempt to get away with it? Athletes do not ask to be role models — should they be free to choose their path towards sporting success? It has been suggested that everyone should be allowed to take performance-enhancing drugs and then see who the winner is. There are several strong reasons to support the legalisation argument.

Many banned substances are not illegal — they are available over the counter. An athlete can use a drug for normal medical care only to find that they are later accused of cheating. This happened to British skier Alain Baxter in 2002. Baxter later cleared his name but was still stripped of his Olympic bronze medal after failing a drugs test as a result of using a nasal inhaler cold remedy. Lots of nutritional supplements contain banned substances, which are not always apparent on the labels, as do cold cures and decongestants, which often contain stimulants. If properly monitored, many of the substances do not pose a health risk. The ease of access to some performance-enhancing drugs may remove another deterrent from the act of taking them.

The testing process itself faces many difficulties. With new drugs (and new masking agents) continually being developed, sports testing programmes face problems keeping one step ahead of the scientists. Note that the drugs themselves are developed for purely medical reasons, but illegal uses are found for them. The testing programmes also face difficulties in gaining access to athletes during training, particularly when at training camps abroad.

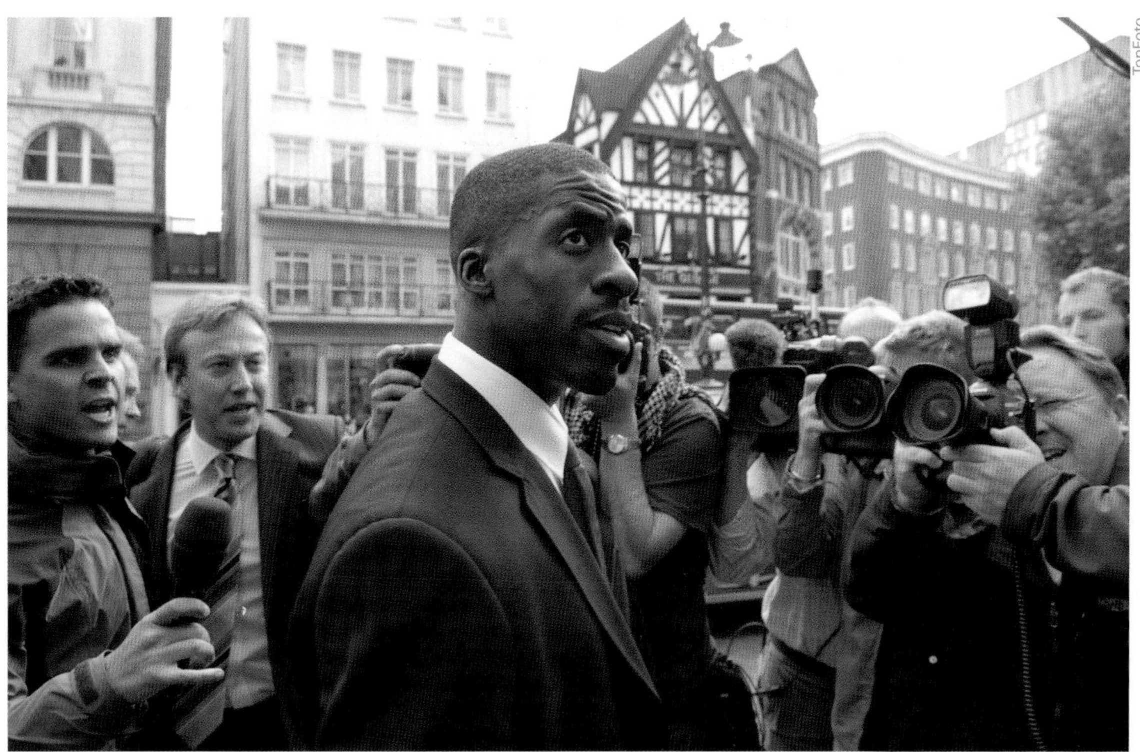

Dwain Chambers at the Royal Courts of Justice in July 2008, to challenge his Olympic ban. The ban was upheld.

The millions of pounds spent annually on testing, and on associated legal cases, could be spent elsewhere. In many cases, testing has proved unsound, jeopardising athletes' careers while others get away with it. The 800 m Commonwealth gold medal-list Diane Modahl was banned from competition in 1994 when tests found she had high levels of testosterone in her urine. Modahl took 2 years to clear her name. An appeal panel accepted that bacterial activity could have altered the sample while it was unrefrigerated.

In addition, there have been legal problems with imposing an outright ban on guilty sports performers. Different countries and different sports have different

Top tip

There are lots of useful websites that provide information on drugs in sport:
www.uksport.gov.uk — site of UK Sport as the agency in the UK responsible for promoting ethically fair, drug-free sport
www.wada-ama.org/en/ — official website of WADA
www.didglobal.com — UK Sport's drugs information database
www.debatabase.org — International Debate Education Association; lots of discussion on topics in the world of sport, including drugs
www.dailydose.net — subscribe to the *Daily Dose* to receive a daily update of drugs in sport news

regulations, which further complicates the issue. British sprinter Dwain Chambers involved UK Athletics and the British Olympic Association in expensive court cases in 2008 in an attempt to overturn his lifelong ban on competing in the Olympics after taking illegal hormones in 2002. Britain is one of the few nations that uphold a lifetime Olympic ban on those found guilty of taking illegal drugs.

Most people, however, feel that the fight to discourage drug-taking in sport should continue. Possible strategies that could be used to prevent drug taking include:

- random and out-of-competition testing
- better coordination between organisations such as **WADA**, UK Sport and NGBs, as well as unifying governing body policies
- campaigns and education programmes for coaches and athletes encouraging ethically fair, drug-free sport, such as UK Sport's 100% Me!
- stricter punishments, such as lifetime bans and the removal of Lottery funding if tested positive
- investing more money into rigorous testing programmes with better technology
- using both positive and negative role models

Despite the efforts of agencies such as WADA and UK Sport, drug taking in sport continues.

Key term

World Anti-Doping Agency (WADA): a partnership of governments and sports organisations attempting to standardise anti-doping programmes worldwide.

Tasks to tackle 14.2

Outline a case for a total ban on the use of drugs in sport under the following headings:

(a) Reasons for a ban

(b) Problems with implementing the solutions

Sport and the law

The deviant acts of performer violence, hooliganism and drug taking are all against society's norms and values and are therefore increasingly likely to attract the attention of the law.

Sport and the law have traditionally been considered as separate areas of life as they have rarely overlapped. However, the number of deviant acts within sport appears to have increased, or it may be that incidents have been more widely reported by the media. In addition, the level of professionalism and commercialisation involved in sport has led to a stricter adherence to legal standards. Thus, the authorities have been forced to make sport as accountable as other social and business institutions.

The needs of various groups, including performers, officials and spectators, should be considered in relation to sport and the law.

Professional performers

Performers have long accepted the 'contract to compete' and have understood the activity they participate in by abiding by its rules. However, the number of prosecutions due to violent acts has risen. Duncan Ferguson (1995) was the first professional soccer player to be imprisoned for an on-the-field assault (head butting a Raith Rovers player while at Rangers). More recently (in 2007), Joey Barton — at the time a player for Manchester City — received a suspended sentence for a training ground assault.

Top tip

Foul play may result in compensation claims.

Performers are employees and as such can be said to have the same employment rights as other workers. In 1995, Jean Marc Bosman, a Belgian footballer, forced the authorities to address the issue of players' rights to play the game in any European country. The European Court of Justice recognised in this case that there was no reason why professional sports players should not enjoy the benefits of the single market, and in particular the free movement of workers, resulting in the abolishment of transfer fees and opening national competitions to players throughout Europe. Players at the end of their contracts can now move on free transfers to other clubs, earning highly lucrative financial deals for themselves as no transfer fee is involved.

Performers seek success, sometimes unethically by the use of banned substances. What sanctions should they face? What rights do athletes such as Dwain Chambers have to appeal against the laws of an organisation such as the British Olympic Association? Some people may feel that the right to appeal against sporting organisations goes against the true ethics of sport, but it is entirely permissible within the British legal system.

Officials

Referees have been prosecuted for allowing situations to occur that have caused permanent damage to a performer. The implications for referees, many of whom are voluntary and amateur, are considerable.

Physios/surgeons

Legal action may be taken due to incorrect treatment of injured performers. In March 2007, footballer Michael Appleton was awarded £1.5 million in damages after judges found that a poorly conducted knee operation cut short his career.

Spectators

Supporters' behaviour has also caused a considerable amount of concern in legal circles. Hooliganism in the 1970s and 1980s brought into question the ability of football clubs to regulate the behaviour of their supporters. Various pieces of legislation have emerged to try to control fans, including:

- the Football Offences Act, 1991
- the Public Disorder Act, 1991
- the Football Spectators Act, 1989

Health and safety

Sports participants have a right to expect facilities and equipment to be properly maintained in order that their health and safety is ensured. This applies to recreational performers as well as elite performers. If accidents occur due to negligence, legal action may result. Such cases have also occurred in school outdoor and adventurous activities (part of the physical education curriculum), and have consequently deterred many teachers from conducting any school trips involving such activities.

Tasks to tackle 14.3

Give reasons for the increased involvement of the law in the protection of elite performers during their sports careers.

Practice makes perfect

1 Give reasons why elite performers may become violent on the field of play. *(2 marks)*

2 What has been done to make football stadiums safer and to prevent and control violence by spectators at football matches? *(4 marks)*

3 The twenty-first century continues to see sports performers resorting to the use of banned drugs to improve performance. Discuss possible methods that could be used to more effectively deter the use of performance-enhancing drugs. *(4 marks)*

Chapter 15 Sport and commercialisation

Evaluating contemporary influences

What you need to know

By the end of this chapter you should be able to understand the advantages and disadvantages of:

- commercialisation
- sponsorship
- the media
- technology

in modern-day sport.

The relationships between sport, the media and business

Sport, the **media** and business are closely inter-linked — the 'golden triangle' — they all influence and affect each other. The media use sport to gain viewers or readers and hence to increase advertising revenue. In turn, the media are used by business organisations to advertise their products. Businesses often pay large sums of money to gain access to the huge consumer audience that views major sporting events. The money earned through sports **sponsorship** and media deals, and through the increased fan base brought by the media, funds better facilities, improved coaching and talent programmes and, ultimately, a greater number of elite performers. World Games, in particular, cost vast sums which commercial interests help to cover.

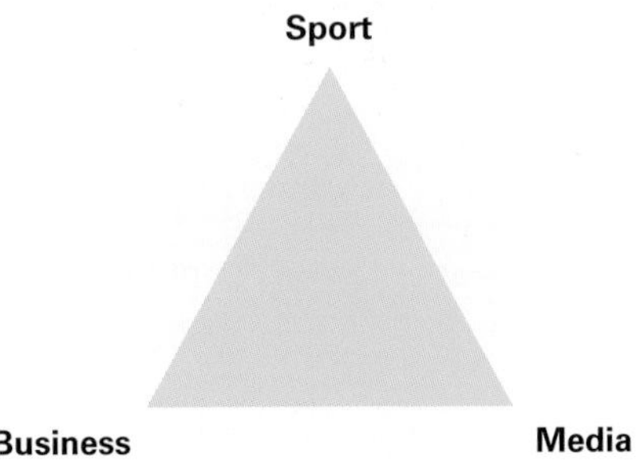

Figure 15.1 The 'golden triangle'

Key terms

Media: newspapers, magazines, radio, television and the internet.

Sponsorship: to support a person, organisation or activity by giving money, encouragement or other help in exchange for favourable publicity or a commercial return.

Commercialism: an emphasis on the principles of commerce, with a strong profit motive.

Commercialisation

As we saw in Chapter 13, the commercial development of sport initially occurred in the nineteenth century as spectator sports emerged. Prior to this, sport was often a locally organised, low-capacity pastime. The massed population needed entertaining and sport was used as a means of achieving this. This was seen by some as an opportunity to organise regular sporting events, which they could make money from. Promoters and agents emerged, and **commercialism** became an important part of sport.

Today, sport is a global product and is marketed around the world. There is extensive media interest in certain 'high-profile' sports, with television companies paying huge amounts of money to gain the right to show a sporting event, for example Premiership football on Sky Sports and Setanta, and hence gain access to a large and lucrative audience.

Commercial sport:

- is professional, high profile and high quality
- becomes a spectacle or display for spectators as part of a mass entertainment industry
- goes hand in hand with sponsorship, business and contracts
- treats athletes as commodities, with a view to increased sales and profits for the companies involved
- is associated with a high level of all forms of media coverage

The impact of commercial, in particular media, interests in sport is so great that the very structure of games has changed to accommodate them (see pages 166–67).

The impact of sponsorship

The exposure on offer from such media coverage leads to sponsorship deals. Sports clothing and equipment firms, such as Nike and Adidas, pay large sums to sponsor teams and individuals to aid their merchandising. Merchandising is also practised by the teams themselves, and even NGBs. Teams, and in some cases individual players, become lucrative brands in their own right, selling everything from team shirts to computer games and washing powder.

Gambling plays an important role in the commercial aspect of sport. New technology, such as internet betting, has led to major gambling websites increasing their role as sport sponsors.

The impact of sponsorship deals on the behaviour of individual performers is important. Think of the racing driver who changes into a baseball cap featuring the sponsor's logo before standing on the podium, or the snowboarder who immediately removes his/her board at the bottom of the run to reveal the board company's logo. Both of these actions are timed to coincide with television close-ups and photo opportunities.

NGBs, agents and commercial ownership

In nineteenth-century Britain, sport was controlled and organised by many small governing bodies. The middle and upper class men who made up these governing bodies tended to favour the amateur code — i.e. a code of fair play and playing 'for the love of it' rather than winning.

In the late twentieth century, many of the governing bodies had to embrace the commercial world in order to compete in modern-day sport and continue to attract top performers into their sport. Bureaucracy may have increased, but it can also be said to have brought more efficient management and business techniques to the sporting world. Nevertheless, as media coverage nationalised and then globalised sport, its organisation became controlled by fewer, richer and more powerful individuals and firms. Rupert Murdoch and his media empire (which includes BSkyB), for example, have great power in media sports coverage. Nike and Adidas, as global competitors in the sport and leisure world, wield vast power in merchandising and sponsorship.

Governing bodies and other organisations have become multinational companies. America's National Basketball Association (NBA) and National Football League (NFL), for example, spread influence and products around the world, including countries such as the UK where their respective sports are not widely played.

There are few opportunities for NGBs to use the media to promote more minority sports. Nations hosting the Olympics, however, are able to include 'demonstration games' in sports for which no medals are awarded but which may be included in the official programme in future.

In order to negotiate the increasingly commercialised world of elite sport, players' employment contracts and sponsorship deals become controlled by managers, or agents, seeking the 'best' for their clients. However, that 'best' may be in terms of financial gain rather than the overall interests of the player. In top-level football, for example, the transfer of a player from one club to another can be negotiated between the agent and clubs without a great deal of input from the player himself, and often involving intense media speculation. All of which may, in turn, affect that player's performance and, of course, future.

Performers and commercialisation

These factors have led to many sports people having limited control over decisions about their careers. This is particularly true of high-profile performers who — as described above — can be owned, contracted and sold with little input. In the 2007–08 football season, striker Carlos Tevez was transferred from West Ham to Manchester United amid complicated bureaucratic wrangling that seemed to marginalise the player himself.

High-profile performers do receive a large income for sports participation and the associated commercial activities. We should not forget that commercialisation is responsible for the professional status of most sports. In order to maintain their commercial status, however, high earners need to deliver high standards of performance on a regular basis. When the rewards are great, and can only be maintained by winning, winning becomes ever more important. The Lombardian ethic of winning at all costs becomes more evident among top-level performers. Athletes can be put under pressure to take risks, for example to perform when injured or to dive to claim a penalty, particularly if they are the main attraction.

In effect, such high-profile performers become public commodities. They are effectively entertainers who become household names: Tiger Woods, Rafael Nadal, David Beckham. Commercial deals tend to focus on image, with personality and looks being as important, if not more so, than talent. Not only must they specialise in a sport in order to compete, which requires serious training, dedication and self-sacrifice, such performers must also be seen to 'act appropriately'.

Commercial sport provides high-profile positive role models, which can lead to increased participation in sport — important in an increasingly inactive and unhealthy society. However, certain sections of the British media, i.e. the tabloid press, know that more papers can be sold when role models are brought down. High-profile performers therefore also suffer from a lack of privacy as the media intrude into their private lives in an attempt to sell papers. When a performer's actions do not live up to the high standards required, a 'media frenzy' may well ensue.

The media

The influence of the media is embedded in the process of commercialisation. It brings with it many advantages, but can be seen as a double-edged sword even for those sports that are deemed as media friendly.

Table 15.1 The advantages and disadvantages of being a media-friendly sport

Advantages of media coverage for a sport	Disadvantages of media coverage for a sport
Raises the profile of the sport Raises the profile of individual players Raises participation levels through positive role models (e.g. tennis during Wimbledon fortnight) May lead to more fixtures and more variants of the game, which further fuels a high profile and high participation levels Increases commercial opportunities, which raises more money for players, facilities, coaching and training opportunities Helps to raise standards of performance through positive role models	Control shifts from the performers and NGBs to agents and television companies Timing, frequency and structure of the game may be adapted to suit the television format Ticket prices increase, which risks alienating some fans Certain prestigious sports events are only available to satellite and cable viewers, which risks alienating some fans (e.g. live international cricket dominated by Sky) Some players become negative role models as increased stakes, including media hype, encourage deviant behaviour

The impact of media coverage on sport formats and organisation

For some sports, the attention of the media has led to fundamental changes in the rules and structure of the game:

- Rules have been introduced to speed up the action to prevent spectator boredom. For example, the multi-ball system in football matches cuts down on time waiting for the ball to be retrieved.
- Changes have been made in the scoring of sports to create more excitement. For example, a bonus league point is now awarded in rugby for scoring four or more tries (introduced at the rugby union World Cup in Australia in 2003); 5 points are now awarded for a try in rugby union (changed from 4 points in 1992); badminton now scores on every point (changed in 2006 from previous scoring rules where you scored points only on your own serve).

- Breaks are provided in play so that sponsors can advertise their products. American Football, for example, is played in four 15-minute sections, with a longer break at half time.
- Competition formats have changed. 20/20 cricket is shorter than the traditional version of the game and has proved a major revenue earner through increased numbers of spectators leading to television and commercial interest. There is concern that it will overshadow other forms of the game including 5-day test matches.
- Timings of matches have been altered to suit television. Premiership football, for example, is often spread from Saturday to Monday evening rather than all matches taking place on the traditional Saturday afternoon. Season structure may also be changed. The Rugby League Conference, for example, was formed in 1997 to play matches in summer, completely contrary to the traditional winter season. Note that such changes can impact on the ability of some fans to follow their team and are not always to the benefit of performers.

Which sports lose out and why?

The globalisation of sport through media coverage can raise awareness of different sports. American football, for example, initially had late-night coverage on Channel 4, but has since moved to the (richer) Sky Sports channel and been promoted via NFL games at Wembley. American football has many media-friendly qualities: it is high-profile, elite, male, able-bodied and structured in short bursts of play to maximise advertising revenue.

By contrast, some sports lose out and receive none of the advantages listed in Table 15.1 above. The result is a loss of profile, lack of funding, lack of role models and low participation levels — all of which further increases the inequality between sports.

There are characteristics that many non-media sports share:

- Lack of mass following by the public. A sport with a small participation base may be deemed to be 'minority' or unfashionable. Some sports have a historically poor following in the UK. The Tour de France, for example, is hugely popular throughout mainland Europe but not historically popular here. Coverage is consigned to ITV3 and the Eurosport channel.
- Seen as less accessible to wider society. Not many people can afford a horse and so are unlikely to experience show jumping, for example. (Note that although very few people can drive a Formula 1 car; most people have a car of some kind.)
- Difficulty in understanding how a winner is found, for example low scoring games or complicated scoring systems.
- Few/no role models for the public to relate to. Can you name a British hockey player?
- The extended nature of a competition may mean it is difficult for an audience to maintain its interest.

Tasks to tackle 15.1

(a) List the characteristics of various sports that make them attractive for television coverage.

(b) Why is test cricket not as 'telegenic' (i.e. appealing to television audiences and producers) as 20/20 cricket?

- Seen as lower status. This label is often ascribed to female and disabled sport. Gymnastics, for example, is generally considered as a female sport. Outside of the Olympics, and despite the presence of role models such as Beth Tweddle, British gymnastics lacks television coverage.

Media technology

Do modern television and broadcasting technologies give the same spectating experience as actually attending the sport event?

On the one hand, high-quality sound and picture technology gives users an impressive view of the sport. Improved media technology, particularly with the introduction of digital television, allows for highly individualised experiences. Viewers are now able to choose the way they experience sport, for example by selecting camera angles (stump cam in cricket), watching more than one match at a time, or listening in to radio links on board with Formula 1 drivers such as Lewis Hamilton.

In many ways, the inclusion of expert commentary and close-up visuals can be said to give media viewers a heightened experience of sport. Action replays and freeze frames allow more detailed analysis of key incidents to take place. On the other hand, viewers' experiences are largely shaped by the commentators and pundits, with little room for alternative views.

Live screenings and 'big screens' can also make a collective experience possible without attending the actual event. On the other hand, media viewing can be said to lack 'real' atmosphere, with little sense of being a part of the spectacle or of playing a role within the contest. There is little interaction with other spectators (for the same team or the opposition) if viewed at home.

Lynne Cameron/Rangers FC/PA Photos

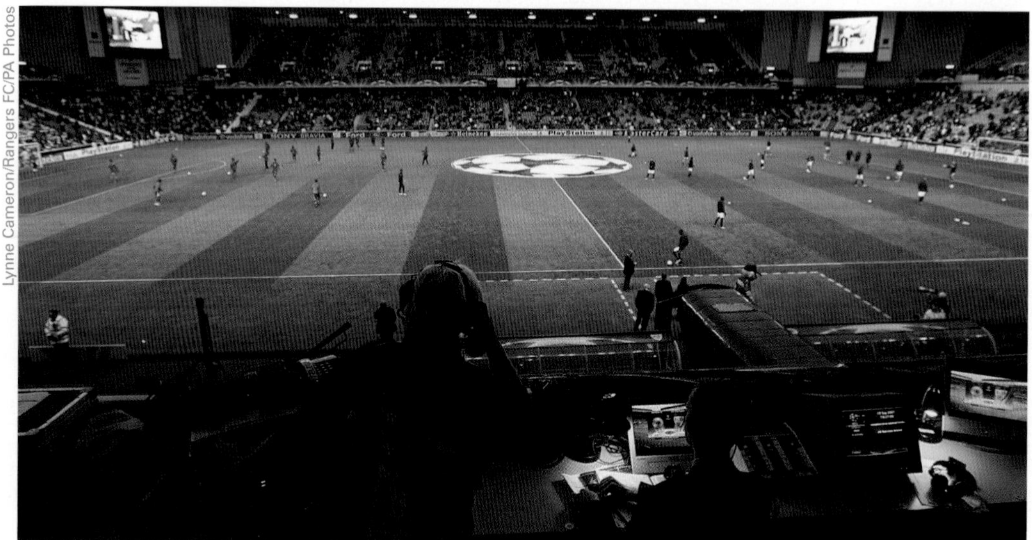

Expert commentary can educate viewers and enhance their viewing experince, especially with action replays. It may, however, present a biased view of the action.

Sports technology: case studies

Sports technology is increasingly used to support the development of UK sports performers. In February 2008, a new £15 million state-of-the-art Sports Technology Institute was opened at Loughborough University and has been involved in the development of personalised football boots for Premiership players, as well as working with Nike and Umbro on next-generation garments for England's rugby and football teams. (See www.sports-technology.com for more details of the Institute's work in a range of different sports.)

The impact of Hawk-Eye

What is Hawk-Eye?

Paul Hawkins designed Hawk-Eye with sport in mind, but not quite knowing where his gizmo might be used. Hawk-Eye has developed as a computer linked to 'on-court' cameras in all major tennis championships. These cameras use infrared beams to make a billion calculations on every point in order to rule on line calls. Hawk-Eye has been in development since the 1980s. The 2007 Artois Championship at Queens was the first grass court tournament to use the technology. It made its debut at Wimbledon on 25 June 2007 on Centre and Number 1 courts.

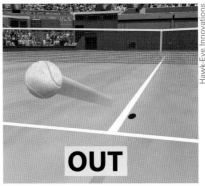

Hawk-Eye Innovations

Tennis Hawk-Eye in action

The use of the technology has led to a new rule in the game: the 'three-challenge' protocol. Players can call on Hawk-Eye to make as many successful challenges to line calls as they want, but only three unsuccessful challenges per set (plus one more for a tie-break).

How has Hawk-Eye been received?

Most players, officials and spectators appear to love Hawk-Eye. It takes the sting out of contentious line calls, so helping to improve relations between players and officials, while also providing an extra element of entertainment/drama for the crowd as everyone awaits the computer's verdict.

There have been some 'teething problems'. Power cuts during the 2007 Queens Tournament put Hawk-Eye temporarily out of action; an inaccurate graphic shown on television caused confusion at the Australian Open in the same year. It has also led to a need to educate both players and spectators about why the marks left by tennis balls (particularly visible on clay courts) do not necessarily prove whether a ball was in or out.

Disadvantages may include the decreased likelihood of eyeball-to-eyeball confrontations between player and umpire, for which John McEnroe was renowned. There have also been accusations of 'gamesmanship', when players use a challenge to take a breather or to unsettle the rhythm of an opponent's play.

Hawk-Eye is also used in cricket and snooker, and is being looked at for football and basketball. Whatever the sceptics say, Hawk-Eye is likely to stay and expand into other sports arenas.

Swimsuits: a help or a hindrance?

Recently, sports technology has been linked to dramatic performance improvements in swimming. At the World Short Course Swimming Championships in Manchester in April 2008, 18 world records were broken in the 5 days of competition. During the championships, FINA — the world governing body for swimming — announced that the Speedo LZR Racer Swimsuit, the centre of the controversy about technology and performance, was legal and met all FINA's stipulated specifications for swimsuits. This announcement included making a clarification on the point that the rules do not limit the fabrics and material used.

This opened the door for other companies, like Arena, to use polyurethane to reduce drag and compress the muscles to apparently create a sensation of buoyancy. More records are likely to fall, benefiting performance standards and creating both crowd and media interest in successful swimmers at global sporting events such as the Olympics and World Championships.

Most spectators would prefer the best swimmer to win whatever suit he/she was wearing. If the breaking of world records is more a result of technological developments in swimwear rather than pure performance improvements, then this may deflect from the ultimate achievement of breaking a world record.

Technology and coaching/officiating

As with Hawk-Eye, new technological developments frequently have implications for coaches and officials. The digital imaging software Dartfish, for example, allows a frame-by-frame analysis that coaches can use to fine-tune performance and eliminate technical errors.

Following some controversial judging at the Beijing Olympics 2008, it was announced that Taekwondo would be using an electronic protector system and video replays at the 2009 World Championships as well as at London 2012. Video replay systems will allow immediate correction of 'incorrect decisions'. This will relieve pressure on officials, as well as ensuring that there is more consistency in officiating and therefore enabling the right person to win. This in turn helps with performer and spectator confidence in the sport.

Tasks to tackle 15.2

How have performers and spectators benefited from advancements in sports technology?

Practice makes perfect

1 Discuss the following statement:
'Modern television and broadcasting technologies can give the same spectator experience as actually attending the sports event.' *(4 marks)*

2 How might media coverage and the commercialisation of sport affect the 'performer' as well as the 'nature of a sport'? *(6 marks)*

3 Identify some possible negative effects of sponsorship for the performer as well as for the sponsors themselves. *(4 marks)*

Unit 4

Optimising practical performance in a competitive situation

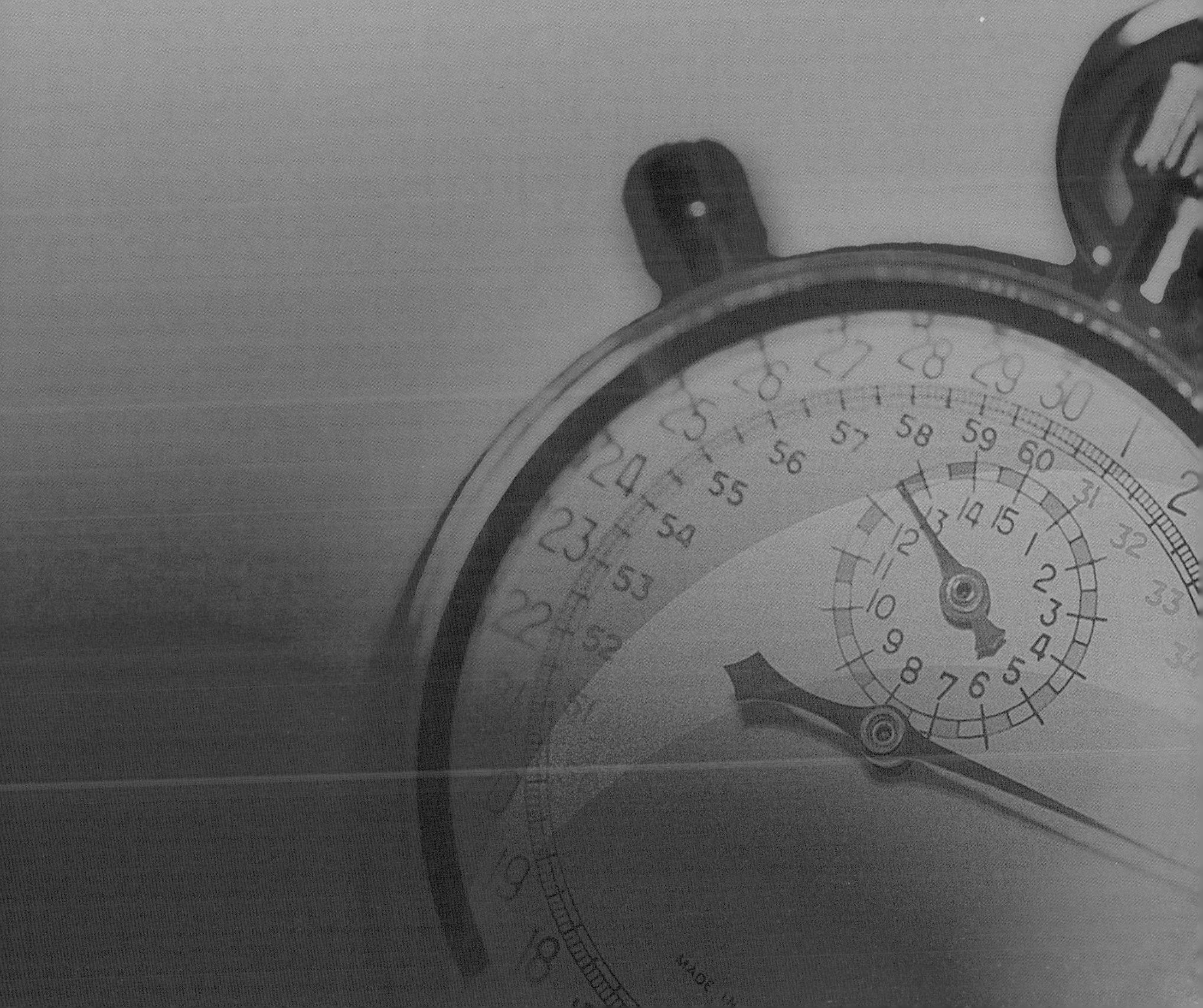

Chapter 16 Optimising practical performance in a competitive situation

Coursework

The A-level coursework unit, Unit 4, is designed to build upon your AS work on roles and performances. From the two roles and activities followed at AS you are advised to optimise your performance in one of them. However, if you feel you would like to choose a totally different role or a different activity, it is entirely up to you — there is no exam board compulsion to stick to the focus of your AS work.

When choosing your one role/activity to undertake at A2, it is important to bear in mind the way you will be assessed. The marking is different from AS, with performance worth half the marks and an evaluation/correction of weaknesses worth the other half.

Top tip

You should choose an activity that you feel you can perform well in your chosen role, as well as understand in relation to its important technical, physical and psychological demands.

In Unit 4 you will be assessed in three different sections:

- Section A — Practical performance
- Section B — Observation, analysis and critical evaluation
- Section C — Application of knowledge and understanding to optimise performance

Section A: Practical performance

This section is worth 60 marks, or half of your A2 coursework.

You will be assessed on your ability to perform in relation to the assessment criteria in one of the following three roles:

- a practical performer
- an official (not in mountain walking)
- a sports leader/coach

As a practical performer, 60 marks can be earned for your performance in a fully competitive game or performance situation demanding more of you than at AS. Example performance situations include a 15-a-side rugby union game, a three-day mountain walking expedition or a trampoline routine. Your performance should therefore involve progression from AS, which was more about core skills in isolation or conditioned situations.

The 60 marks available can be earned as follows:

- **Area of assessment 1** — technical quality aspect/event 1: attacking (or equivalent as stated by the activity criteria in the specification)
- **Area of assessment 2** — technical quality aspect/event 2: defending (or equivalent as stated by the activity criteria in the specification)
- **Area of assessment 3** — application of strategies and tactics to optimise performance in the chosen activity

Top tip The three areas of assessment are worth 20 marks each.

In order to gain as many of these 60 marks as possible it is important that you are physically fit enough to meet the demands of your chosen activity, for example playing for 90 minutes in football without too much fatigue, running 5000 m without losing technique, performing a gymnastics routine from start to finish with as few mistakes as possible. It is also important that you are at the optimum level of psychological arousal so that you can concentrate while performing to the highest level possible.

If you choose to act as a leader or coach for an activity, the 60 marks are divided into three similar sections to those of the performer described above. However, as a leader/coach you will be assessed on your ability to communicate with performers and prepare them physically and psychologically as appropriate to the performance situation facing them. If as a leader/coach you notice any areas which can be improved in the performer(s) you are working with — for example in relation to their physical, psychological and decision-making capabilities — then it is important to identify them, explain them to the performers and correct them as appropriate so that performance standards rise.

Should you choose the role of official at A2 you will be expected to officiate in a fully competitive situation and illustrate your understanding of such a role before, during and after the event. Suitable examples include umpiring a netball match and judging starts and turns during a swimming gala. It is important to ensure safe and fair competition for the participants you are officiating. Suitable preparation, for example studying official national governing body rule books, is important to enable you to demonstrate understanding of the rules and scoring systems in the activity you are officiating and application of them during live performance. While assessment areas 1 and 2, linking to technical quality, are similar to those of a performer/coach, assessment area 3 is slightly different. As an official, this requires you to communicate with the performers and other officials present. You will need to be able to justify your decisions, keep a record of scoring and ensure safe practice throughout. There is, of course, also the requirement to equip yourself as necessary to officiate in your chosen activity.

Section B: Observation, analysis and critical evaluation

This section is worth 30 marks overall. Sections B and C can be completed as either written pieces of work, verbal interviews or a combination of interview and written work (which is probably the best option).

Identification of weaknesses

First, you need to analyse and critically evaluate your own performance as a performer or official, or the performance of another named coach if you are acting as a leader/coach, compared with the skills assessed in the sport and role chosen. The identification of performance weaknesses is worth 15 marks.

Comparison with an elite performer

To complete Section B, you then need to compare these weaknesses with the performance of an elite performer, official or coach as appropriate to the role chosen. This is worth 15 marks.

When completing both parts of Section B, it is important that you link your comparisons to the three areas of assessment completed in Section A, i.e. technical quality aspects 1 and 2, and assessment area 3. The quality of your response to each of your identified weaknesses will be marked out of 5, so it is important to give the same amount of detail to all parts of your work. When comparisons are made to perfect technical models (elite performer, coach or official), they need to be directly linked to what you do not do quite as well. The following examples are taken from the Category 1 Performer Activities listed in the specification:

- Aspect 1 — attacking (football performer). Link to areas such as the technique of different shots, crossing a ball, performing attacking headers.
- Aspect 2 — defending (basketball performer). Link to areas such as the defensive stance position, rebounding, ability to perform in a zone defence and/or man-to-man systems.
- Area of assessment 3 — strategies and tactics (tennis performer). Link to areas such as shot selection in a rally, movement of opponent around the court, when to attack from the net and when to stay on the baseline.

Section C: Application of knowledge and understanding

This section is worth 30 marks overall. You need to make sure that you identify causes of the weaknesses that have been identified in Section B (15 marks).

When considering the causes of the weaknesses identified in Section B it is important to explain them clearly. One way of doing this is to divide your work into three clear sections that link to technical aspects 1 and 2, and assessment area 3.

Weaknesses in attacking technique may link to decision making and fitness components. Weaknesses in the ability to rebound successfully in basketball or to achieve greater height in the high jump could link to a lack of power and subsequent decrease in performance in comparison with the named elite performer.

Finally, appropriate corrective measures should be explained for the weaknesses identified. This will require you to apply relevant parts of theory covered at both AS and A2. For example, you might list appropriate methods from anxiety control from Unit 3 if you have identified over-anxiety prior to competition as a weakness for a swimmer or athlete. Similarly, you might list appropriate methods of stretching from your Unit 2 work if lack of flexibility is a cause of weakness for a gymnast.

Top tip

The key to success with Sections B and C of the A2 coursework is relevance to your chosen sport or role rather than simply including as much theory as possible that bears little significance to the weaknesses identified.

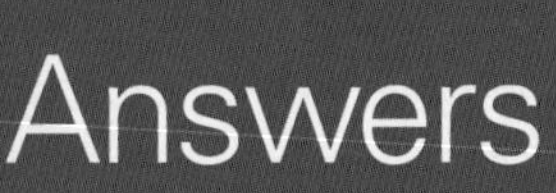

Answers

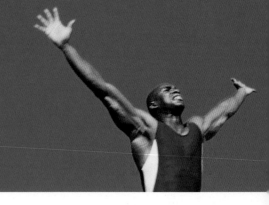

Tasks to tackle

Chapter 1

1.1 (page 5)

Activities that predominantly use the ATP-PC system are high intensity, lasting longer than 3 seconds but no more than 10 seconds. Examples include a 100 m sprint, a short rally in tennis, a full court press in basketball, or a short sprint for a through ball in football.

1.2 (page 9)

Name of game	ATP-PC system	Lactate anaerobic system	Aerobic system
Football	A short sprint lasting longer than 3 seconds, e.g. to get free to receive the ball	A sprint lasting longer than 10 seconds, e.g. when on a break from the defensive half to the attacking half	Positional play when the intensity is low and the duration is more than 3 minutes

2.1 (page 13)

Factor	Change
Temperature	Increases
ATP stores	Decrease
Phosphocreatine stores	Decrease
Glycogen stores	Decrease
Triglyceride stores	Decrease
Carbon dioxide levels	Increase
Oxygen/myoglobin stores	Decrease
Lactic acid levels	Increase

2.2 (page 15)

Examples of ways to delay a game by 30 seconds: a time-out, fake an injury, kick or hit the ball as far away as possible so someone has to go and get it! There are many sport-specific answers.

4.1 (page 25)

Slow twitch (type I)	Fast twitch (type IIa)	Fast twitch (type IIb)
Marathon runners	800m runners	Sprinters (100m and 200m especially)
Swimmers	1500m runners	Throwing event specialists
Distance runners	Gymnasts	Weightlifters
Triathletes		
Cross-country skiers		

5.1 (page 32)

Supplements	
Endurance athlete	**Power athlete**
Glycogen loading	Creatine monohydrate
Herbal remedies	Herbal remedies
Protein supplements	Protein supplements

Ergogenic aids	
Endurance athlete	**Power athlete**
EPO	Anabolic steroids
HGH	HGH

6.1 (page 37)

Off-season — rest and general fitness

Pre-season — a lot of intensive fitness training

Competitive season — maintenance of fitness and skills training

6.2 (page 39)

Training aim	Details of training session
A session to improve lactate tolerance	This needs to be a session that works the lactate anaerobic system, e.g. interval training. The athlete completes a work interval of 200m at 90% max heart rate followed by a 90-second rest interval. This should be repeated six times, followed by a 5-minute rest and then another set.
A session to improve strength in the upper body	Weight training exercises, e.g. shoulder press, lateral pull downs, lateral raises, biceps curls, triceps extensions

8.1 (page 46)

Newton's laws	Application
Law of inertia	Any sporting example where the state of motion of either the ball or the body changes, e.g. a rally in tennis when the ball changes direction
Law of acceleration	Any sporting example where the force applied is proportional to the rate of change of momentum, e.g. more force is required for a smash
Law of reaction	Any sporting example where the action force is equal to the reaction force, e.g. a jump

8.2 (page 49)

(a) Displacement: swim = 1.5 km, bike ride = 0 km, run = 200 m

(b) The average speed and the average velocities for the components of the triathlon:

Distance	Time	Displacement	Average speed	Average velocity
1.5km (1500m) swim	30min 30 (1830s)	1.5km (1500m)	0.82ms^{-1}	0.82ms^{-1}
40km (40000m) cycle	90min (5400s)	0.0km (0m)	7.41ms^{-1}	0.0ms^{-1}
10km (10000m) run	45min (2700s)	0.2km (200m)	3.7ms^{-1}	0.07ms^{-1}

8.3 (page 50)

(a) Any three examples when acceleration or deceleration may be important: to lose a player, to beat an opponent, to get to the ball first, to create momentum etc.

(b)

Distance (m)	0	20	40	60	80	100
Velocity (m s^{-1})	0.0	8.5	11.1	11.5	11.5	9.5
Time (s)	0.0	2.9	5.6	7.6	9.4	11.4
Acceleration	N/A	2.93	0.96	0.20	0.00	–1.00

8.4 (page 50)

Performer	Mass (kg)	Velocity (m s^{-1})	Momentum (kg m s^{-1})
100 m sprinter	80	10.0	800
Prop	105	8.5	893
Centre forward	70	9.5	665
Middle-distance runner	65	9.0	585

8.5 (page 52)

(a) Where the force is being applied (point of application)

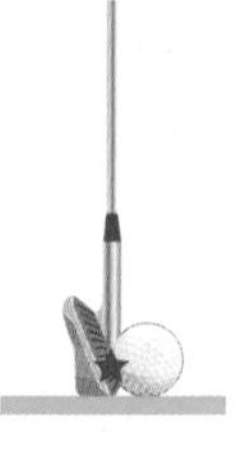
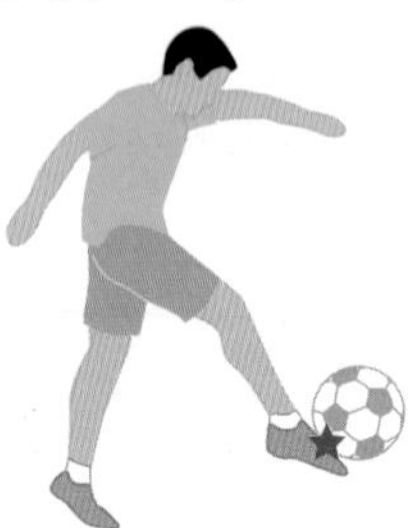
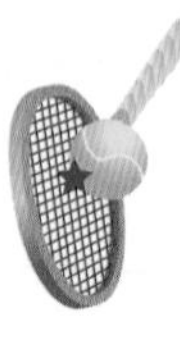

(b) Direction of the force

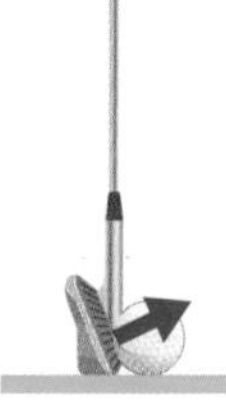
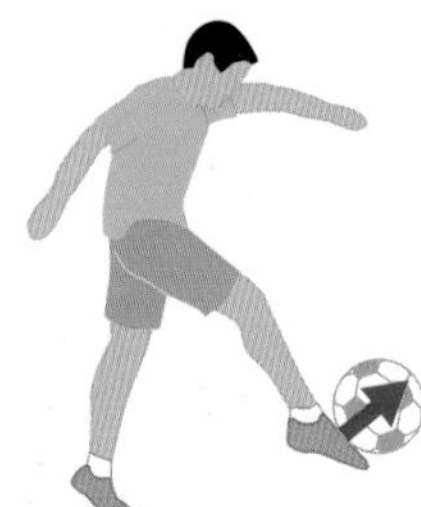
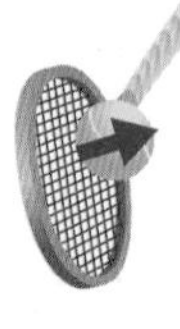

(c) Size of the force

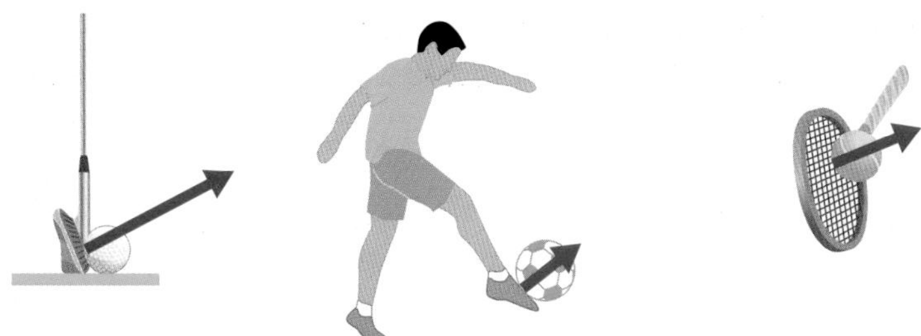

8.6 (page 56)

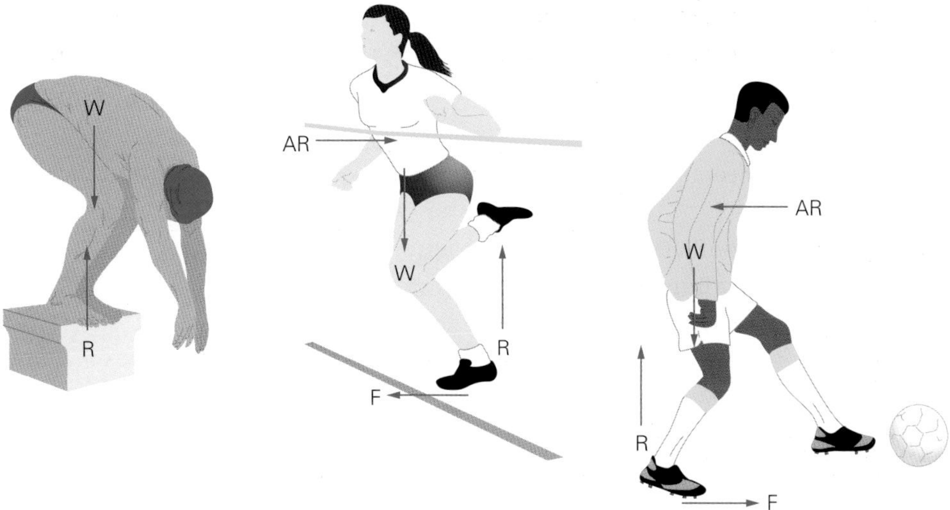

8.7 (page 60)

Any three sporting examples when a force is applied outside the centre of mass — for example, free kick to curve the ball, top spin in tennis, spin bowling in cricket.

9.1 (page 69)

At least one point in each category.

Method	Advantages	Disadvantages
Questionnaire	Quick Deals with lots of information Cheap Objective	Biased answers Socially acceptable answers Misunderstand question
Observation	True to life	Subjective Observer needs training
Physiological	Factual Can make comparisons	May cause stress Restrictive to players, therefore not used in real game

9.2 (page 73)

Cognitive: beliefs — any example showing a belief in exercise or training to improve health, well-being or fitness, e.g. you believe in the health benefits of going to the gym.

Affective: feelings — any example to show enjoyment of physical activity, e.g. you enjoy a football training session.

Behavioural — any example to show physical actions and participation, e.g. you go to football training twice a week.

9.3 (page 77)

Freedom of expression is allowed here to show any aspect of aggression. It should include, for example, the factors that cause aggression — instinct, frustration, learned cues, social learning.

10.1 (page 81)

Forming — meeting up and getting to know the others in the team and their roles and personalities
Storming — conflict and tension as rivalries are encountered
Norming — settling down as differences are resolved
Performing — working together to try to achieve goals and results

10.2 (page 82)

Judgement can be used here to produce a list of answers. The important thing is that you can recognise the difference between task and social cohesion. Suggestions include:

- type of sport — task cohesion
- leadership — task and social cohesion
- past/future success — task cohesion
- coordination — task cohesion
- social loafing — task and social cohesion

10.3 (page 88)

There are many examples of suitable leadership styles for differing situations:

- autocratic — danger or team that is unsure of themselves
- democratic — with a small group
- rewarding — with beginners
- social support — with an individual after a defeat
- training and instruction — leading up to a major game to improve performance
- laissez faire — with experts

11.1 (page 91)

Performance accomplishments — set easy goals, allow early success, point out past success

Vicarious experience — show role models of same age and ability successfully doing the task; give accurate demonstrations

Verbal persuasion — use positive feedback, positive reinforcement; give encouragement

Emotional arousal — control anxiety with relaxation techniques and imagery; use positive self-talk

11.2 (page 93)
Any goals that show steps towards success, including both process and performance goals that are short term, before the long-term objectives are met. For example, a tennis player might improve her service technique (process), then make a greater percentage of successful first serves in each game (performance) to improve her ranking (long term).

11.3 (page 100)
Causes of anxiety include being watched, increased competition such as a big game, frustration, conflict, evaluation apprehension. For example, being watched by a county selector during a trial game.

11.4 (page 110)

Locus of causality

Locus of stability	Internal	External
Stable	**a**	**d**
Unstable	**c**	**b**

12.1 (page 114)
The word 'discuss' is more likely to be seen at A2 than at AS and involves writing answers pointing out the positives as well as the potential negatives of a given issue.

Positives/benefits of hosting 2012:

- improve facilities and regenerate area
- economic benefits, such as increased tourism
- increased participation, leading to an increase in health and fitness
- feel-good factor; increase in national pride
- social inclusion

Negatives/drawbacks of hosting 2012:

- relocation of homes, businesses (sometimes against a person's wishes)
- high costs to taxpayers
- leaves debt
- increased security risk
- normal life disrupted due to increased visitor numbers
- legacy of expensive, sometimes unused, facilities (if legacy is not part of overall strategic plan)

12.2 (page 120)

Policies Sport England has developed to encourage increased participation in sport. Choose three from:

- Sport Unlimited
- Free swimming initiative for under-16s and over-60s
- Extending Activities
- Whole Sport Plans
- Activemark, Sportsmark, Sports Partnership Mark
- PESSYP
- Coaching for Young People

12.3 (page 123)

Summer Olympic investment, 2006–09 (£)	
Athletics	20 378 000
Rowing	20 049 000
Cycling	17 494 000
Swimming	16 699 000
Hockey	8 573 000
Triathlon	3 897 000
Table tennis	2 219 000
Weightlifting	1 437 000

12.4 (page 130)

UK Sport is influencing the development of sports excellence in the UK in a number of different ways. Choose from:

- oversight of UKSI
- promotion of ethically fair and drug-free sport (e.g. 100% Me!)
- distribution of Lottery funds to the elite via World Class Performance Pathways
- runs the World Class Events programme

12.5 (page 132)

NGBs support and develop performers at elite performance levels. Choose from:

- talent identification schemes

- selection of performers for World Class Performance Pathways/SportsAid/TASS funding
- give access to high-level facilities and equipment
- train high-level coaches in their sport
- provide sports science support
- organise and provide information about competitions

13.1 (page 137)

Characteristics of rational recreation are summarised below.

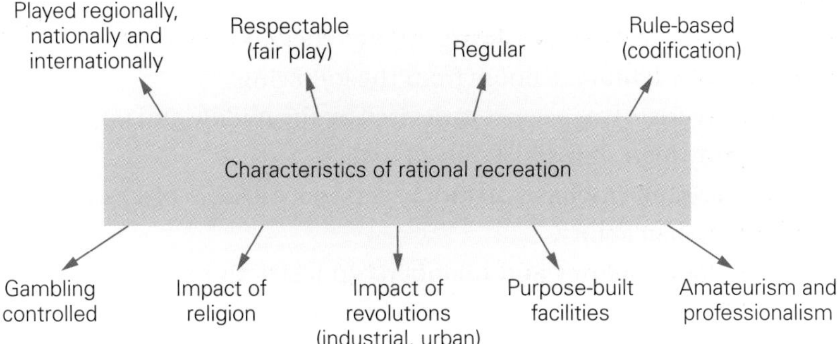

13.2 (page 138)

Popular recreation	Rational recreation
(1) Local	(1) Regional/national
(2) Few rules	(2) Codified
(3) Cruel/violent	(3) Respectable
(4) Occasional	(4) Regular
(5) Rural	(5) Urban
(6) Natural resources	(6) Purpose-built facilities

13.3 (page 142)

(a) The 'half day' Factory Acts influenced sporting development at the end of the nineteenth century by increasing the time available for workers to play and/or watch sport. Saturday was half-day closing at factories and so sports, particularly football, were played on a Saturday afternoon.

(b) Sociocultural factors influencing the rational development of sport in late nineteenth-century Britain. Choose four from:

- travel and communications (railways) — improved accessibility for sport
- emergence of urban middle class — factory teams, facilities provided
- urbanisation — purpose-built facilities in limited space
- church — provided facilities and set up teams
- time — gradual increase in free time (e.g. Saturday afternoons off)

13.4 (page 146)

Features of amateur athletics during late nineteenth-century Britain. Choose from:

- strict class divide evident
- middle class keen to stay exclusive
- competed for intrinsic rewards/self challenge
- working class keen to earn money
- middle/upper class formed their own clubs and established NGBs (AAC in 1866; AAA in 1880)

13.5 (page 147)

(a) Reasons for amateurs having higher social status than professionals in the nineteenth century. Choose from the following:

- Amateurism was a concept devised by the middle and upper classes. They were already high status in a classed society.
- It placed an emphasis on moral/personal qualities of sport, giving these higher status than ability.
- Exclusion clauses and membership restrictions were designed to keep out members of the working class who were seen as low status.
- There was a direct link between public schools, universities and NGBs, allowing power to be maintained.

(b) The effects of social class for an elite level performer in early twentieth-century Britain: It was easier for members of the middle/upper class to become elite performers as they had time and money. Lack of time and finance restricted working class development.

To begin with, working-class professionals were only allowed to participate in certain sports and in specified roles. The middle/upper classes used restrictive membership clauses/policies to deny outsiders access to the majority of sports. The 'amateur code' of participation excluded working-class athletes financially and socially for many years, into the twentieth century.

13.6 (page 148)

Violence could be seen as outside the 'contract to compete', as it:

- deprives the victim of a fair chance to try to win
- is against the ethics/rules of an activity
- is against the law

But in some sports, 'violent acts' are within the rules and are therefore 'acceptable', e.g. ice hockey (body checking), boxing etc.

13.7 (page 149)

(a) G, **(b)** C, **(c)** S, **(d)** S, **(e)** C, **(f)** G

14.1 (page 156)

Violence among players can be caused by: frustration with the score or officials; emotional intensity surrounding a particular match; crowd provocation; provocation by an opponent; conflict within a team; the lack of a suitable deterrent.

Violence among spectators can be caused by: frustration with the score or officials; pre-match media hype or traditional rivalry; provocation by opposition supporters; poor deterrent (poor policing); alcohol and drugs; organised violence; copying violence on the pitch.

14.2 (page 160)

(a) Reasons for a ban: drug taking is immoral/unfair; it is illegal; endangers health; sets a poor example; lowers the status of sport/a particular sport.

(b) Problems with implementing the solutions: difficulties in testing successfully and prosecuting offenders; still worth the risk for athletes due to high rewards for success; increased costs associated with improving tests; difficulties in accessing performers.

14.3 (page 162)

Reasons why elite performers may need protection from the law during their careers:

- compensation claims, e.g. against the opposition for foul play resulting in long-term/career-threatening injuries
- contracts with employers
- deals with sponsors
- protection from media intrusion into private life
- appeals against NGB disciplinary decisions/drug tests
- protection from racism
- protection from violent fans

15.1 (page 167)

(a) Sports that are attractive to television:

- demonstrate high levels of skill
- demonstrate competition (opponents are potentially well matched)
- demonstrate aggression/physical challenge
- have reasonably simple rules/scoring systems
- fit into a relatively short timescale
- show role models/well-known personalities
- have national relevance/traditionally part of our culture (e.g. football/cricket in England)

(b) Test cricket matches:

- are mostly played during the 'working day' (20/20 is at night/weekends)

- last for 5 days, which makes it difficult for some to maintain interest (20/20 is over in a few hours)
- feature action that is too slow or technical for most viewers (the rules of 20/20 lead to all-action entertainment)
- may be perceived as traditional/boring (the coloured clothing/'razzmatazz' of 20/20 makes it more attractive to individuals of all ages)

15.2 (page 170)

Benefits to performers from advancements in sports technology:

- Advancements in clothing can improve training/performance (e.g. Speedo sharksuits).
- Tailor-made equipment can be designed to performers' preferences (e.g. Premiership players' football boots).
- Faster rehabilitation/injury recovery (e.g. oxygen tents/hyperbaric chambers).
- Improved feedback on performance (e.g. frame-by-frame analysis).
- Increased knowledge of diet/sports supplements.

Benefits to spectators from advancements in sports technology:

- Increased sense of crowd involvement (e.g. Hawk-Eye appeals carried out live and on-screen for fans to see).
- Improved experience of watching sport at home through more cameras.
- Improved excitement if top-level performances/world records result from improved technology.

Practice makes perfect

Chapter 1

1 Fats; fatty acids; glycerol; triglycerides *(up to 2 marks)*
Carbohydrates; glycogen; glucose; protein/lactate *(up to 2 marks)*
(3 marks in total)

2 Any six for 6 marks:

- during low-intensity exercise, 50% of energy comes from fats and 50% from carbohydrates
- as the intensity increases, less fat is used and more carbohydrate is used
- at high intensity, carbohydrates are the only energy source, with no fats being used
- at low intensity, fats and carbohydrates are broken down using oxygen (aerobically)
- fats require more oxygen for breakdown
- mitochondria/Krebs cycle
- at high intensity, fat use is limited by oxygen availability, as no fats can be used anaerobically

- energy release from fats is slow, while there is a quick release of energy from carbohydrates
- glycolysis
- lactate formation

3 The 100 m runner uses the ATP-PC system/phosphocreatine system/alactic system. *(1 mark)*

Any three for 3 marks:
- PC is stored in muscles.
- PC = C (creatine) + Pi (phosphate) + energy
- Energy is used for ATP regeneration.
- ADP + Pi + energy = ATP (ADP + PC = ATP + C)
- ATP is broken down into ADP + P + energy.
- The process is anaerobic (no O_2).

(4 marks in total)

Chapter 2

1 The 800 m swimmer is breathless due to EPOC/excess post-exercise oxygen consumption. *(1 mark; no marks for 'O_2 debt/deficit')*

Any three for 3 marks:
- aerobic energy needed
- requires oxygen (O_2)
- restoration of PC/ATP/phosphagens
- resaturation of myoglobin with oxygen
- lactate/lactic acid breakdown/removal
- high temperature/high metabolic rate
- energy for high heart rate/breathing rate

(4 marks in total)

2 A = alactacid/fast component
B = lactacid/slow component
(2 marks)

3 Any four for 4 marks:
- lactic acid used as energy source/using oxygen (O_2)/lactate to replenish ATP
- oxidised into carbon dioxide (CO_2) and water
- in inactive muscle and various tissues/organs
- converted to glycogen/glucose
- then stored in the liver
- some is excreted in sweat/urine/conversion to protein

Answers

Chapter 3

1 VO_2 max is the maximum oxygen uptake/consumption/used *(1 mark)*; per minute/unit of time *(1 mark)*.

2 Any five for 5 marks:
- increased maximum cardiac output
- increased stroke volume/ejection fraction/cardiac hypertrophy
- greater heart rate range
- less oxygen being used for heart muscle, so more available to muscles
- increased A-VO_2 diff
- increased blood volume and haemoglobin/red blood cells/blood count
- increased stores of glycogen and triglycerides
- increased myoglobin (content of muscle)
- increased capillarisation (of muscle)
- increased (number and size) of mitochondria
- increased concentrations of oxidative enzymes
- increased lactate tolerance
- reduced body fat
- slow-twitch hypertrophy

3 Any three for 3 marks:
- lactate threshold is when lactate begins accumulating in the blood/onset of blood lactate accumulation/OBLA
- when fitter, lactate threshold is delayed; occurs at a higher level of energy/workload/%VO_2; elite/fitter performers can tolerate higher levels of lactate or equivalent
- because fitter people can remove lactate more quickly/produce less
- lactate can be converted to protein/glucose/glycogen/CO_2 and water
- lactate as an energy substrate for aerobic energy

Chapter 4

1 Fast-twitch (glycolytic) fibres/type IIb *(1 mark)*
Any five characteristics for 5 marks:
- fast motor neurone conduction velocity
- large muscle fibre diameter
- low number of mitochondria
- low capillary density
- low myoglobin content
- high PC stores
- high glycogen stores
- low triglyceride stores

- fast contraction/relaxation time
- high force production/more powerful
- easily fatigued

(6 marks in total)

2 Any four for 4 marks:

Fast-twitch:

- have faster contractions/twitches/faster (myosin) ATPase
- have more PC
- fatigue easily
- have more glycogen
- have fewer mitochondria
- have less myoglobin
- have lower oxidative capacity
- have more force/strength/powerful contractions
- have larger motor neurone/(motor) unit/fibre diameter

3
- motor unit consists of motor neurone/nerve *(1 mark)*
- and muscle fibres *(1 mark)*

Any three for 3 marks:

- number of motor units used can vary
- size of motor units can vary
- all or nothing law
- spatial summation/timing
- fast-twitch motor units produce more force/slow-twitch produce less force
- repeated nervous stimulation without time to relax
- this produces stronger contractions in the motor unit
- wave summation

(5 marks in total)

Chapter 5

1 Any three for 3 marks:

- Endurance athletes require more carbohydrates than power athletes.
- Because they exercise for longer periods of time/need more energy.
- Proteins are very important for power athletes.
- Proteins are important for tissue growth and repair.
- Endurance athletes may manipulate their diet/use glycogen loading.

2 Any three for 3 marks:

- EPO
- An increase in the oxygen-carrying capacity of the body

- leads to an increase in the amount of work performed.
- Can result in blood clotting/a stroke/in a few cases, death.

3 **Creatine**

Advantages:

- It allows the ATP-PC system to last longer.
- It helps to improve recovery times.

Disadvantages:

- Side effects could be dehydration/bloating/muscle cramps/slight liver damage.
- Most ends up in urine rather than in the muscle.

(2 marks max)

Sodium bicarbonate

Advantages:

- It allows the performer to continue to exercise at a very high intensity for longer.
- It increases the buffering capacity of the blood so it can neutralise the negative effects of lactic acid.

Disadvantages:

- It can cause vomiting/pain/cramping/diarrhoea/a bloated feeling.

(2 marks max)

(4 marks in total)

Chapter 6

1 Any four for 4 marks:

- training divided into sections/stages for a specific purpose
- macrocycle — a long-term goal
- mesocycle — a period of training lasting weeks/months on a particular aspect
- microcycle — a week of training sessions
- dividing the training year into competitive phase/peaking/tapering/playing
- pre-season training
- out-of-season recovery

2 Any three for 3 marks:

- ratio of carbon dioxide produced to oxygen consumed
- referred to as the respiratory quotient (RQ)
- determines which energy source is being oxidised
- RER value between 0.7 and 1.0 = a mix of carbohydrate and fat
- RER value of approx 0.8 = protein
- RER value greater than 1.0 = anaerobic respiration

3 Any three for 3 marks:
- when an eccentric contraction is performed
- this stimulates the muscle spindle apparatus/detects the stretch
- which sends a nerve impulse to the central nervous system (CNS)
- the CNS initiates a stretch reflex, causing a powerful concentric contraction as the performer jumps up
- as a result, more overload/power can occur

Chapter 7

1 Any three for 3 marks:
- DOMS is the delayed onset of muscle soreness
- performer may experience tender and painful muscles some 24–48 hours after exercise
- muscle soreness occurs as result of structural damage to muscle fibres and connective tissue surrounding the fibres
- as a result of excessive eccentric contractions
- which occur mostly during weight training and plyometrics

2 Any three for 3 marks:
- The aim of hyperbaric chambers is to reduce the recovery time for an injury.
- The chamber is pressurised/increases the amount of oxygen that can be breathed in.
- As a result, more oxygen can be diffused to the injured area.
- The dissolved oxygen can reduce swelling and stimulate the body's cells to repair.
- Such chambers are often used by performers to speed up the recovery time of broken bones.

3 Any three for 3 marks:
- The performer should remain in the ice bath for 5–10 minutes.
- The cold water causes the blood vessels to tighten and drains the blood out of the legs.
- On leaving the bath, the legs fill up with new blood containing oxygen to help cells function better.
- The blood that leaves the legs takes away with it the lactic acid that has built up during the activity.
- Ice baths are now used by most professional sportsmen and women who train and play regularly.

Chapter 8

1 Any six for 6 marks:
- First law of motion/law of inertia. A body remains in a constant state of motion unless acted upon by a force.

- The high jumper applies a force to change his/her state of motion from the run-up to the take-off.
- Second law of motion/law of acceleration. The magnitude/size of the force governs acceleration at take-off/change of momentum.
- The direction of force controls the direction of acceleration.
- The more force that is applied, the more height results.
- Third law of motion/law of action and reaction. To every force there is an equal and opposite reaction force.
- The ground reaction force needs to generate a large vertical component for the high jump.

2 Any two for 2 marks:

- vectors have magnitude/size
- vectors have direction
- a point of application
- a line of application

(up to 2 marks)

Any three for 3 marks:

- A force is applied to the ground by the contraction of muscles.
- An equal and opposite reaction force moves the performer/ground reaction force produces the movement.
- Vectors have vertical and horizontal components.
- The sprinter requires a large horizontal component.
- The high jumper requires a large vertical component.

(3 marks max)

(5 marks in total)

3

- impulse = force × time/*Ft*
- and equates to change in momentum

(up to 2 marks)

Any two for 2 marks:

- constant mass
- impulse has direction
- single footfall
- positive impulse is needed for acceleration at take-off
- negative impulse occurs when foot lands/breaking action
- if net impulse is positive, acceleration occurs

(2 marks max)

(4 marks in total)

4 Any six for 6 marks:

- ice is friction-free surface
- angular momentum remains constant during rotation
- angular momentum = moment of inertia × angular velocity
- moment of inertia = spread/distribution of mass around axis
- angular velocity refers to speed of rotation
- change in moment of inertia leads to change in angular velocity/speed of the rotation
- bringing arms closer to body/axis of rotation = increase in angular velocity
- taking arms further away from body/axis of rotation = decrease in angular velocity

Chapter 9

1 Any three for 3 marks:

Trait theory states that characteristics of personality:

- are innate/born with them/inherited
- are stable/consistent behaviour/same in most situations
- are enduring/last a long time
- can be used to predict behaviour

2 Any four for 4 marks:

A negative attitude can be changed into a positive attitude by:

- using persuasion/persuasive communication
- (persuasion is more effective if given by an expert)
- cognitive dissonance/challenge beliefs
- showing positive role models of similar age and ability
- making activities fun/varied training
- pointing out health benefits

3 Any four for 4 marks:

Aggressive tendencies can be reduced by:

- using relaxation techniques
- using cognitive techniques, such as imagery or mental rehearsal
- using channelling to change aggression into assertion
- walking away from the situation/calming down/counting to ten
- punishing aggressive acts/substituting the player
- reinforcing non-aggressive acts in training
- setting non-aggressive goals

Answers

Chapter 10

1 A group has interaction *(1 mark)*, a common goal *(1 mark)*, an identity *(1 mark)*.

2 Any five for 5 marks:

- A prescribed leader is from outside the group.
- An emergent leader is from within the group.

Leader characteristics include:

- charisma
- empathy
- motivation
- communication skills
- experience

3 (a) Potential productivity is the group's best possible performance *(1 mark)*.

(b) Any three for 3 marks:

Influences that produce faulty processes include:

- coordination problems/tactics/strategies
- social loafing
- lack of motivation
- Ringlemann effect

Chapter 11

1 Up to 3 marks for benefits of goal setting:

- improves confidence
- provides motivation
- lowers anxiety
- gives something to aim for/provides target

Up to 3 marks for SMARTER principle:

- specific
- measured
- agreed
- realistic
- timed
- exciting
- recorded
- goals should not just include winning; include performance/process goals as well

(6 marks in total)

2 1 mark for each of the following:

- State anxiety — in a particular situation/temporary
- Trait anxiety — innate/more permanent/consistent

- Cognitive anxiety — psychological/worry/irrational thoughts
- Somatic anxiety — physiological/tension/heart rate

(4 marks in total)

3 1 mark for including mention of Zajonc theory.

1 mark for each of:

- increased arousal
- evaluation apprehension
- dominant response
- better performance or facilitation if task is well learned — dominant response likely to be correct
- worse performance or inhibition if task is new — dominant response likely to be incorrect
- inhibition if task is performed by a novice/facilitation if task is performed by an expert

(7 marks in total)

4 Any six for 6 marks:

Learned helplessness:

- is the sense that failure is inevitable
- is blaming internal and stable reasons for losing
- can be general
- or specific

Learned helplessness can be countered by:

- attributional retraining
- changing internal/stable reasons for failure to external/unstable ones
- giving positive feedback
- redefining failure
- setting easier goals

Chapter 12

1 Any two for 2 marks:

World Games characteristics:

- elite performers — find number 1 in the world
- multi-sport (e.g. Olympics) or single-sport (e.g. World Cup rugby/football)
- promote 'national pride'
- worldwide media coverage/commercial opportunities
- bring different nations together in a spirit of healthy competition

2 Any four for 4 marks:

National institutes of sport develop elite performers by:

- providing a network of local/regional centres for elite performer development

- offering free access to sports centres for elite performers
- national organisation and regional delivery for closer access from home
- providing high-class/top-level training facilities
- providing high-class/top-level coaching
- providing general sports science/medical back-up
- providing Performance Lifestyle Advice (career/educational help and support)
- linking to NGBs and talent identification programmes

3 Any three for 3 marks:
Sports Coach UK is helping the development of sports performers by:
- developing high-level coaches/high-performance coaching programmes
- working closely with NGBs to promote coach education
- developing a coaching award structure
- providing resources/workshops to develop coaches — sold via Coachwise Limited
- coordinating the 'Coaching for Teachers' initiative
- providing a support network of regional Coach Development Officers

4 Any three for 3 marks:
The Lottery is funding sports excellence by:
- funding the World Class Performance Programme/Pathways
- providing money for training, accommodation costs, Athlete Personal Awards
- funding organisations involved in elite sport (e.g. UK Sport, NGBs, EIS etc.)
- funding high-level facilities and equipment
- helping to attract/fund world-class sports events
- helping to fund mass participation schemes and widening the participation base

5 Any two for 2 marks:
Criteria to receive SportsAid funding:
- up-and-coming performers
- with NGB recommendation/potential
- with a proven financial need
- not supported by other sources such as Lottery funds

Chapter 13

1 Changes from mob football to association football linked to:
(a) working conditions:
  - factory system led to regular work times
  - reduction in working week
  - professional football seen as a relatively good job
  - workers had enough money to pay to watch on a Saturday afternoon

(2 marks max)

(b) urbanisation:

- loss of space
- specialist/purpose-built facilities developed
- large numbers in a small area needed positive pastimes

(2 marks max)

(c) transport, i.e. trains and trams:

- allowed regular fixtures
- facilitated development of spectatorism
- required standardised rules

(2 marks max)

(6 marks in total)

2 Any three for 3 marks:

Amateurism and professionalism in the second half of the nineteenth century in football:

- The FA was formed by ex-public schoolboys/amateurs.
- Amateurs were upper class and middle class, while professionals were working class.
- Payments were given to professionals only.
- Violence in professional games increased due to an increased desire to win, with players' livelihoods at stake.

3 Any three for 3 marks:

Gamesmanship means:

- using 'cunning means' to win/stretching the rules to their limit but not actually cheating/breaking the rules
- not following the etiquette of the activity
- deceiving an official
- distracting an opponent (e.g. verbal 'sledging')
- time wasting/delaying play (e.g. in tennis, appealing a decision when you know the ball is 'in' or taking an injury time-out to disrupt the flow of an opponent's play when you are really fit to play)
- pre-match psyching out tactics

4 Any three for 3 marks:

The effects of fair play in a sport/sporting situation:

- helps sports officials as they can focus on making correct decisions
- helps flow of event/game
- increases goodwill among players
- increases goodwill among spectators
- raises status of a sport
- produces positive role models to follow

Answers

Chapter 14

1 Any two for 2 marks:

Reasons for violence on the field of play:

- over-emphasis on winning
- extrinsic rewards at stake
- encouragement to do so (e.g. from the coach)
- loss of control (e.g. retaliation against opponent)
- lack of ethical/moral restraints on personal behaviour

2 Any four for 4 marks:

Ways to prevent/control football hooliganism:

- legislation
- all-seater stadiums
- segregation of fans
- better policing, use of coordinated police intelligence
- control ticket sales (e.g. at fixtures with a previous history of violence)
- use of CCTV to monitor fans/pick out known troublemakers
- tougher deterrents/ban known troublemakers
- ban/control alcohol sales
- increase sanctions on clubs with bad records in football hooliganism

3 Any four for 4 marks:

Methods to use as possible deterrents:

- increase random/out-of-competition testing
- improve international agreements on sanctions/punishments of offenders
- harsher punishments/life bans
- educate performers (e.g. about side effects/morals) of drugs
- improve testing procedures — use of role models

Chapter 15

1 Any two for 2 marks:

Agree:

- enhanced sound and picture quality enhances experiences
- technology allows for more individualised experiences (live screenings/player cam/Hawk-Eye/reffu link)
- can watch as part of crowd/community in pubs/work places

Any two for 2 marks:

Disagree:

- no all-encompassing view/lacks 'true' atmosphere
- experience shaped by the producer/commentator

- little/less sense of being a part of the spectacle/playing a role within the contest
- unlikely to interact with opposition spectators

(4 marks in total)

2 Effects of commercialisation on a performer. Any three for 3 marks:

- may become a public commodity with possible negative effects on private life
- may need to concentrate on image/style/the need to sell oneself to attract sponsorship — which detracts from sports training
- may be encouraged to entertain and to take risks
- performers now high earners/stars/role models

Effects of commercialisation on a sport. Any three for 3 marks:

- NGBs pushed to change the rules to make matches more entertaining/exciting (e.g. 20/20 cricket)
- increases inequality between commercial and non-commercial sports
- timings may be altered to suit television
- the popularity of sport may be enhanced/money in the game for grass roots development

(6 marks in total)

3 Possible negative effects of sponsorship for the performer. Any two for 2 marks:

- possible insecurity — may lose sponsorship if lose form/suffer an injury
- possible exploitation — intrusion into private life/too much of a controlling influence
- inequality — minority sports performers have difficulty getting sponsors
- deviance — temptation to cheat to win

Possible negative effects of sponsorship for the sponsor *(2 marks)*:

- high risk — success of the performer is not guaranteed
- possible low returns — high outlay may not be matched by increased sales

(4 marks in total)

Index

A

acceleration 46, 49, 178
  deceleration and 49
  law of (second law of motion) 45
acetylcholine, reduced levels 12
achievement motivation 71–2
actin filament 26
actual productivity 80
adenosine diphosphate (ADP) 3–4
adenosine triphosphate (ATP) 2–3
Adidas 164, 165
aerobic endurance 37
aerobic exercise 18, 19
aerobic system 3, 6, 7
  advantages and disadvantages 7
affective component 72
  emotional feeling 73
age differences 19
aggression 152
  controlling 79
  in sport 66, 76–9
aggressive cue theory 78
agreed goals 93
air resistance 54, 55, 59
alactacid component 14, 15
altitude training 35
Amateur Athletic Association 146
Amateur Athletic Club (AAC) 146
amateurism 146–48
Amateur Swimming Association (ASA) 145
amino acids 4
anabolic steroids 31, 157
anaerobic energy systems 4
anaerobic glycolysis 5
angle of release 57–8
angular acceleration 61
angular displacement 61, 62
angular motion 59–65
angular velocity 61, 64
anxiety 93–101
Appleton, Michael, footballer, damages 161
Arena polyurethane swimsuits 170
Armstrong, Lance 42
Arnold, Dr Thomas 142
arousal 79
  and performance, relationship 101–5
Arsenal factory team 140
Artois Championship, Queens 169
assertive behaviour 76, 79
Athens, Olympic Games, 2004 113
athleticism 142
athletics 145–46
ATP 3, 15
  regeneration 3, 8
  synthesis, reduced rate 11
ATP-PC system 3, 4–5, 9, 29
  advantages and disadvantages 5
attitude changing 73–6
  predicting behaviour 76
attribute 109–10
attribution theory 109–11
audience, effects of 106, 107
authority 153
autocratic leadership style 85–8
axes of rotation 60, 63, 65

B

balanced tension 152
Bandura's self-efficacy theory 90
Barton, Joey, assault 161
bathing machines 144
Bath, spa town 144
Baxter, Alain, failed drugs test 158
Beckham, David 165
  2002 football World Cup 42
  metatarsal fracture 41
behavioural component 72
  physical response 73
Beijing, China, Olympic Games 2008 113
beta blockers 31, 157
beta oxidation 7
biofeedback 99
bloating, side effect 29
blood
  doping 157
  glucose levels 13
  lactate 22
  measurements 39
  removal rate 22
  pressure 11
  viscosity 12
blood sports, criminalised 139
body
  as 'temple of the Lord' 142
  composition 19
  growth 2

temperature 16, 32, 33
body hair shaving 54
Bosman, Jean Marc, Belgian footballer 161
Botham, Sir Ian 70
Botham, Liam 70
boxers 68
breathing techniques 99
breathing, increase in 16
British empire 142
British Olympic Association 160
broken time payments 141
buffering 22

C

caffeine 30
calcium, reduced levels 12
Cambridge Rules Football 140, 141
Cantona, Eric,
community sentence 152–53
carbohydrates 3
in diet 34
carboloading *see* glycogen loading
carbon dioxide 6
catastrophe theory 102, 104
catharsis 78
central nervous system (CNS) 36
Chambers, Dwain, Olympic ban 159, 161
channelling aggression 79
charisma of leader 85
cheating 145, 153
Christianity 142
Church, influence of 142–43
class structure 139, 140
co-actor 106
cock fighting 139
codification 136
cognitive anxiety 95, 96
control of 96, 97
cognitive component 72
cognitive dissonance 74, 76
cognitive, thought process 73
cohesion 81–4
influences on 82–3
commercialisation 143, 160, 163–66
commercial sport 164
communication skills 85
competition period 38
competition-specific training 37
competitive players 89
competitor 106
concentration 94
conditioning, general 37
confidence in sport 89
confidence raising 84
conflict 108, 152–54
conservation of angular momentum 64
contract to compete 148
Cooper 12-minute run 20
coordination 81, 83
cortisone injections 41
Coubertin, Baron Pierre de 148–49
coupled reaction 4
creatine monohydrate 29
cricket
and Hawk-Eye 169
professional 147
criminally deviant 151
cross-section of moving body 54
crowd violence 154
cue utilisation hypothesis 103
cultural influences 138

D

Dartfish software for coaching 170
Da Silva, Eduardo, broken leg 42
data collection and trait theory 68
deceleration 46, 49, 178
dehydration 11
side effect 29
democratic leadership style 85–8
dendrites 27
deviancy 148, 151, 152
diet
for athletes 33–4
poor 18
disease and pollution 145
displacement 46, 47
distance 46, 47
factors affecting 57–9
distraction conflict theory 108–9
distribution of mass from axis of rotation 63
diuretics 157
dominant response 102
DOMS (delayed onset of muscle soreness) 43–4
Douglas bag 20
drag 54
drive theory 101–2
drug taking 148
physiological reasons 157
psychological reasons 157
side effects 157
social reasons 157
in sport 156–60
drug types 157
drugs-testing process 158–59
duration of activity 2, 8

E

educating performers 153
Edwards, Jonathan 143
efficacy expectations 90
electrolyte balance 32–3
electron transport chain 6, 7
elite performers, support for 112–35
emergent leader 85
emotional arousal 90, 92
emotional control of performance 89–111
endothermic reaction 3
endurance activities 42
endurance athlete 32, 34
endurance performance, successful 20
energy 2, 3
energy continuum 8–10
England cricket team, Ashes win 2006 73–4
enzymes 3

Index

EPOC (excess post-exercise oxygen consumption) 14
ergogenic aids, illegal 31
erythropoietin (EPO) 31
Eton Wall game 141
European Courts of Justice 161
evaluation apprehension 107
excess post-exercise oxygen consumption (EPOC) 14
exciting goals 93
exercise intensity 22
exothermic reaction 3
external reason for winning or losing 109, 110
extroversion, inherited trait 66, 67
extrovert personality 102

F

facilitated performance 107
Factory Acts 142
  'half day' 183
  time off 139
factory football teams 140
fair play 76, 149
  versus winning 164
fast oxidative glycolytic muscle type 24
fatigue
  causes of 11
  offsetting 13–17
  and recovery 11–17
fats 4, 34
  as energy source 7
faulty processes 80
Federer, Roger 66
Ferguson, Duncan, assault 161
Ferguson, Sir Alex 85
Fiedler's contingency model 86
film, *Chariots of Fire* 143
FINA (world governing body for swimming) 170
fines for aggression 79
flexion of arms and legs 63
flight path of shuttlecock 59
Football Association, 1863 139, 141
  'respect' campaign 151
football boots, personalised 169
football hooliganism 154–56
  causes 154–55
  solutions 155
football, laws of motion in 46
Football League, 1888 141
Football Offences Act, 1991 161
Football Spectators Act, 1989 161
force
  application 51
  balanced 55
  mass and 179
  size or magnitude 51
  time and 56, 57
  unbalanced 55
forces affecting projectiles 59
forming stage 81
foul play 79
fractures 41
free movement of players in Europe 161
free time 142
friction and slippage 53, 55
frustration–aggression theory 77, 78

G

gambling 164
  controlled 139
gamesmanship 149, 169
gender differences 19
Gerrard, Steven, metatarsal fracture 41
ginseng 29
globalisation of sport 167
glucose 6
glycogen 3, 34
  breakdown 8
  depletion 11
  levels 13
  loading 30–31
  replenishment 16
glycolysis 5, 6
goal setting 96, 99
  in sport 92–3
Golgi tendon organs 24, 37
gravitational force 53
group behaviour 75
group cohesion 82
group formation stages 81
group integration 82

H

haemoglobin levels 42
Harvard step test 20
Hawk-Eye 169, 170
health and safety 162
health, poor 139
health risks of drug-taking 158
heart monitoring 99
heart rate increase 16
height of release 68
herbal remedies 29
high-profile performers 165
home advantage 108
hooligans 154, 155
horizontal force 53
hormones, increased activity 16
hostile aggression 76–7
human growth hormone (HGH) 31
hydrogen 7
hydrogen ions 11, 12
hyperbaric chambers 41
  recovery method 42
hypotonic drinks 33

I

ice baths 41
  recovery method 43
imagery 96–8
  cognitive technique 79
impulse 56–7
  graphical representation 57
increased arousal 108
industrialisation 142
industrial patronage 140
Industrial Revolution 136, 38–39
inertia, law of (first law of motion) 45–7
  moment of 63

inhibited performance 107
injury, serious 153
instability, neurotic behaviour 67
instinct theory 77
intensity of activity 2, 8
interaction 81
interactionist approach 70–1
internal reason for winning and losing 109, 110
International Olympic Committee (IOC) 158
introversion, inherited trait 66, 67
introvert personality 102
inverted U theory 102, 103, 105

J

junior versions of sports 91

K

Kingsley, Rev. Charles 142
Krebs cycle 6, 7

L

lactate accumulation 22
lactate dehydrogenase 5
lactate sampling 39
lactate tolerance 177
lactic acid 6, 9, 15, 43
  build-up 11
lactic anaerobic system 3, 5
  advantages and
    disadvantages 6
laissez faire style of leadership 87
law and sport 160–62
law of acceleration 177
law of inertia 177
law of reaction 177
leader behaviour 87
leader characteristics 85
leadership 83, 85–88
  factors affecting 87
  skills 69
  styles 85–88
  Chelladurai's model 86, 87
learned helplessness 110–11
legalisation of drugs 158–60
Liddell, Eric, missionary in China 143
lifestyle 18
lifetime Olympic ban 160
Likert scale, on attitudes 76
linear motion 45
  measurements 46
liver damage, side effect 29
locus of causality 109, 110, 181
locus of stability 109
Lombardi, Vince, football coach 148
Lombardianism 152, 165
long-distance runners 12
Loughborough University 169
low-oxygen environment 42

M

macrocycle 37, 38
Malvern, spa town 144
Manchester United 85
  factory football team 140
Maradonna, Diego, Argentine footballer 75
marathon runner 10
Mascherano, Javier, sent off 151
mass 46, 47
mass of object 63
mass versus weight 47
mastery orientation 110–11
match timing changes 167
McEnroe, John 66, 169
measured goals 93
mechanics of movement 45–65
media 163
  coverage 166
  advantages and
    disadvantages 166
  frenzy 166
  influence 75, 166–68
  technology 168
media-caused changes 166
medulla oblongata 13
mental characteristics of athletes 67
mental practice 98
mental rehearsal 96–8
  cognitive technique 79
merchandising 164
mesocycle 37, 38
metatarsals 41
microcycle 37, 38
middle and upper classes 146
mitochondria 6, 7, 8
mob football 141
mob games 139
Modahl, Diane, gold medallist ban 159
moment of force 60
moment of inertia, high and low 63, 64
momentum 46, 50
mood states, profiles 67
morally deviant 151
motivation reduction 84
motor neurone 27
motor unit 27, 28
movement, mechanics of 45–65
multiple unit summation 27
multistage fitness test 20
Murdoch, Rupert, media empire 165
muscles
  contraction 27
  cramp, side effect 29
  fibre type 22, 24–5
  glycogen 34
  hypertrophy 43–4
muscle spindle apparatus 24
muscles, structure and function 23–8
Muscular Christians 142
muscular contraction control 24
muscular endurance 37
muscular relaxation techniques 92
muscular tension 99
myofibril 23, 25
myoglobin 15
myosin filament 26

Index

N

Nadal, Rafael 165
narcotics 157
narrow band trait theory 67
nation building 113
national governing bodies (NGBs) of sport 140, 143–44, 160
nature and nurture debate 78
nature versus nurture in leaders 87–8
need to achieve (NACH) characteristics 71–2
need to avoid failure (NAF) characteristics 71–2
negative deviancy 151, 152
negative moods 67
nerve cells 27
net force 55
net impulse 57
neurones 27
Neville, Gary, metatarsal fracture 41
Newton's laws of motion 45, 62, 64, 177
Nike 164, 165, 169
non-violence 139
norming stage, group formation 81

O

observation of behaviour 68
Olympic Games 37, 112
  athlete's contract 156
Olympic ideal 148–49
onset of blood lactate accumulation (OBLA) 21–2
outcome goals 92
overcrowding 139
overuse injuries 41
Owen, Michael, metatarsal fracture 41
oxygen (O_2) 14, 35
oxygen consumption in sporting performance 18
oxygen tents (hypoxic tents) 41, 42

P

painkillers 157
Paris Olympics gold medal 143
partial pressure of oxygen 35
patronage
  by middle class 140
  of urban middle classes 142
peak flow experiences 105
peak performance 38
pedestrianism 145
peer group pressure 79
perception 93, 94
performance
  accomplishments 89–90
  and arousal 101–5
  goals 92
  identification 84
performance-enhancing drugs 158
performers and commercialisation 165–66
performing stage 81
periodisation 37–9
perpendicular distance 60
personalities of players 83
personality traits 66, 67
phosphocreatine (PC) 3, 4–5, 15, 29
phosphofructokinase (PFK) 5
physical exercise and psychological wellbeing 69
physical practice 98
physical relaxation techniques 79
physical testing 69
physiological adaptations 19
plyometrics 35–6
popular recreation 136, 183
  characteristics 137–38
positive deviancy 151, 152
positive moods 67
positive self-talk 96, 98–9
potential productivity 80
power athlete 32, 34
power in media sports coverage 165
prejudices 74–6
preparation period 37
prescribed leader 85
prevention 42
process goals 92
professional clubs today 143
professional football 154
professionalism 143, 146–48, 160
professional performers 160–61
profile 67
  of mood states (POMS) 67, 68
projectile motion 57–9
proprioceptive neuromuscular facilitation (PNF) 36–7
proprioceptors 24
proteins 4
  in diet 34
  supplements 30
psychological aspects
  optimising performance 66–89
  team playing 80–9
public baths 145
public commodities 165
Public Disorder Act, 1991 161
public school
  backgrounds 146
  games 141
  influence 139, 140
  values 141
punishing violence 153
punishments 160
Puritan-style Sabbatarianism 143
PWC170 cycle ergometer test 20
pyruvic acid 5

Q

questionnaires 68, 69

R

race fixing 145
Radcliffe, Paula 19
railway transport 139
random testing 160
rational recreation 136–43, 183
  characteristics 137–38
reaction force 53, 55

reaction, law of (third law of motion) 45
realistic goals 92–3
real time 98
recorded goals 92–3
recovery process 13
recreation
regional 136–37, 139
regular 136–37, 139
respectable 136–37, 139
rule-based 136–37, 139
recruitment of motor units 27
referee prosecutions 161
referee's role in aggression 79
regeneration of ATP 3
rehabilitation 42
relaxation techniques, progressive 99
release 57–9
religion, influence of Christianity 139
respiratory exchange ratio (RER) 39–40
reticular activating system (RAS) 67, 103
revolutions 139
rewarding style of leadership 86
rewards 83
RICE (rest, ice, compression, elevation) 41
Ringlemann effect 84
role models 70, 73, 91
Rooney, Wayne, broken metatarsal 41
rotating body 62
rotational force, torque 60, 62
rotation, axes of 60
rowing 147
Rugby Football Union 1871 141
rugby league 147
rugby players 68
Rugby School 147
rugby Super League teams 43
rugby union 147
rule-breaking 148
'runner's knee' 41
running contest 145
rural fairs 145

S

sarcomere 25, 26
sarcoplasm 8
satisfactory performance 90
scalar quantities 46
'seaside towns' 144
sedentary lifestyle 18
self-efficacy theory 89–92
self-serving bias 110
shape of moving body 54
Sheppard, Rt Rev. David, Bishop of Liverpool 143
shin splints 41
significant others 70
influence 73
situation affecting leadership 87
skeletal muscle 23
sliding filament hypothesis 25–6
slow oxidative muscle type 24
SMARTER principle for goals 93
smoking 18
snooker and Hawk-Eye 169
Soccer/Association Football 141
'soccer' 140–41
social benefits 145
social cohesion 81
social facilitation 106–9
social influences 138
social integration 113
socialisation 70
social learning theory 69–70, 78–9
social loafing 84
social support style of leadership 86
sociocultural factors 183
sodium bicarbonate 30
somatic anxiety 95, 96
reducing 99
spa movement 145
spa towns 144
specific goals 93
spectatorism 139
spectators' behaviour 161
speed 46, 48
of rotation 64
versus velocity 48
Speedo sharksuits 186
Speedo LZR Racer Swimsuit 170
spin 64
sponsorship 113, 163, 164
sport
commercialisation and 163–75
deviance and 151–62
entertainment 163–64
law and 151–62
origins of 136–50
rationalisation: case studies 144–46
sport competition anxiety test 100
sporting clubs 140
sporting ethics 136–50
sporting icons 70
sporting image, negative 158
sports clothing sponsors 164
sports injuries 41–4
sportsmanship 149
sports performer, individual influences 66–79
sports psychologists 67
sports supplements 29–34
Sports Technology Institute 169
sports technology, case studies 169–70
stability, consistent behaviour 67
stable extrovert 67
stable reason for winning or losing 109, 110
state anxiety 99–100
state confidence 89
stimulants 157
stimuli, frequency of 27
storming stage 81
strength training 35–6
stress 79, 93–101
stress response 94
stressors 94
success 83

Index

Summer Olympic
investment 182
supporters 106
surface of moving body 54
sweating 11–13, 32–3
swimming 144
swimsuits 170

T

tabloid press 166
Taekwondo video replay
systems 170
tapering 38
task cohesion 81, 82
team cohesion 84
team dynamics 80–1
team games 10
team playing 80–8
team sports and coordination 83
team work 69
technology in sport 163
temperature regulation 12
tennis championships 169
'tennis elbow' 41
testosterone in urine 159
Tevez, Carlos, footballer 165
thermoregulation 12
thermoregulatory centre 13
thought stopping 96, 99
timed goals 93
tissue repair 2
torque, rotational force 60, 62
total momentum 50
Tour de France 2007, drugs 158
training 22
and instruction style of
leadership 87
and muscle fibre type 25
preparation of body 32–4
training unit 38–9
training, specialised 35–40
trait anxiety 99–100
trait confidence 89
trait theory 66–70
travel by railway 139
triadic model 72
triglycerides 4
tropomyosin 26
troponin 26
television advertising 167, 168
Type A and Type B
personalities 67

U

UK Athletics 160
UK Sport 160
UK Sport 100% Me! 160
Umbro 169
unstable reason for winning or
losing 109, 110
urban festivals 145
urbanisation 138–39, 142

V

vector quantities 47, 51
velocity 46, 48
of moving body 54
of release 59
verbal persuasion 90, 91
vertical force 53
vicarious experience 90, 91
video technology 153
violence 160–61, 184, 185
control of 141
drunkenness and 143
spectators 154–56
sports performers 152–54
visualisation 96–7
VO_2 max
evaluation of 20, 21
factors affecting 18, 19

W

wagering 145
Wash House Acts (1846–48) 145
washing facilities 145
water
balance 32–3
importance of 32–3
weight 46, 47, 59
of vertical force 53, 55
optimal 33
Wiener's model of attribution 110
Wilkinson, Jonny, self-talk 98
Wimbledon 169
'win at all costs' 148, 152
winning or fair play 164, 165
Woods, Tiger 165
working classes 147
sport for 139
working hours 142
World Anti-Doping Agency
(WADA) 160
World Cup 1986 75
World Games and elite
performers 112–35
advantages and
disadvantages 14
impact 113–14
World Short Course Swimming
Championships 170

Z

Zajonc theory 195
Z line 26
zone of optimal functioning
(ZOF) 104–5